DOING NEUROFI
AN INTRODUCTION

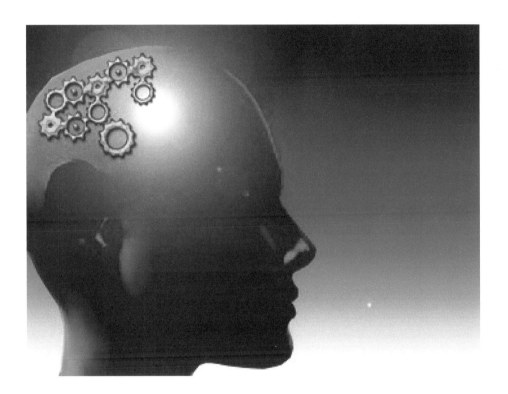

RICHARD SOUTAR, PhD
ROBERT LONGO, MRC

THE ISNR RESEARCH FOUNDATION

EMAIL: CYNTHIA@ISNR.ORG

2011 ISNR Research Foundation
1925 FRANCISCO BLVD. E. #12
SAN RAFAEL, CALIFORNIA 94901
CYNTHIA@ISNR.ORG

PRINTED IN THE UNITED STATES OF AMERICA

ISBN: 978-0-9846085-4-6

COVER ART: CYNTHIA KERSON, PHD

CONTACT THE AUTHORS:
RICHARD SOUTAR, PHD
DRS@NEWMINDCENTER.COM
ROBERT LONGO, MRC
ROBERTLONGOLPC@GMAIL.COM

CONTENTS

LIST OF DIAGRAMS*

*All images are public domain or designed by the author(s) except for those noted within the text

LIST OF TABLES

Chapter 1: History and Perspectives in NFB and QEEG

Quantitative electroencephalography (QEEG)[1] and neurofeedback (NFB) training (also referred to as EEG biofeedback, neurobiofeedback, and neurotherapy) are fields in the early stages of development. QEEG and NFB are practiced by a variety of innovators and professionals from diverse fields who have come together to contribute their expertise to the growth of both areas. Nonetheless, QEEG and NFB enjoy a distinct and unique history.

To truly understand these fields is to comprehend the many competing theories regarding what NFB does to the brain, the disorders it helps, and the best way to employ it. At this time, NFB is still considered experimental in many respects, and practitioners should never make claims of curing a particular disorder. Additionally, the length of treatment varies among patients. NFB usually takes 20-60 sessions on average. Some patients attain results with fewer than 20 sessions, while others may require in excess of 60 sessions for treatment to be effective. When patients reach their treatment goals, an additional 5-10 sessions are often conducted to help set in (consolidate) the NFB training.

QEEG has become more standardized, but there are still several techniques, models, and methods used to gather QEEG data. As professionals, we cannot use QEEG as a diagnostic tool; however, QEEG can help support established or suspected diagnoses. Therefore, it has a differential diagnosis value. Periodic QEEG, or retesting patients once NFB has begun, helps to reassure neurotherapists that NFB is having the desired effect. Most recently, QEEG has been held up as a valid reliable measure of testing in the New York District Court as cited below.

Court Upholds Use of QEEG by Non-physicians in Expert Witness Testimony

In what amounts to a landmark decision, particularly for quantitative EEG (QEEG) and neurofeedback practitioners, a New York District Court judge has ruled that expert witness testimony based on QEEG evaluations meets what is called the Daubert standard. Daubert is a legal precedent set in 1993 by the Supreme Court regarding the admissibility of expert witnesses' testimony during federal legal proceedings. It essentially states that trial judges, as "gatekeepers" of scientific evidence, must determine if expert witness testimony is "relevant" and "reliable."

Daniel Kuhn, M.D. of New York made the case for QEEG and Neuroguide-based interpretations in an affidavit presented to the Court, assisted by Bob Thatcher, Ph.D. The judge's decision in this case also noted that expert witness testimony using QEEG was not the sole domain of neurologists, indicating that other professionals are qualified to testify as QEEG experts. Dr. Kuhn has tracked the progress of this case and posted

---

[1] The term *quantitative electroencephalography* has been abbreviated as both qEEG and QEEG. For

additional information on his website, www.kuhncenter.com under Forensic Services, Frye hearing. [2]

This chapter provides a brief overview of the history and development of QEEG and NFB. A more detailed history of the field can be found in *Mindfitness Training* by Crane and Soutar (2000) and *A Symphony in the Brain* by Robbins (2000). A list of similar titles and recommended readings is located at the end of this book. The experts discussed in this chapter have each had a profound impact on the field.

NFB EXPERTS

Richard Canton

Richard Canton was the first to discover changes in the brain's electrical activity in animals after mental activity occurred and is considered a leader in biofeedback (Criswell, 1995; Demos, 2005).

Hans Berger

In 1924, Hans Berger (born in Neuses, Germany) measured EEG on the human scalp. He was the first to record raw EEG tracings (changes in electrical potential measured between two electrodes placed on the surface of the head) on paper. Berger established the Berger rhythm, 10 Hz alpha, and characterized the resultant wave patterns, including alpha and beta waves. His findings were published in 1929.

Wilder Penfield

Wilder Penfield, a Canadian neurosurgeon, was the first person to do brain mapping in 1928. Penfield worked with patients who suffered from epilepsy. Before operating on patients, he measured the motor cortex and discovered various sites of movement. Penfield stimulated the different parts of their brains with electrodes to locate the cells that set off their attacks while the patients were awake. He learned exactly where each part of the body that was being touched or moved was represented in the brain. Penfield's work became known as homunculus *("little man")*, and his sensory map was depicted in cartoons of the somatasensory and motor areas.

Herbert H. Jasper

Herbert Jasper developed a standard set of electrode placements on the scalp, so that results obtained in different clinics and laboratories could be compared. This standard set became known as the 10-20 International System.

According to Patent Storm:

> In 1949, Jasper's work was adopted for trial at the General Assembly of the International Federation meeting held in Paris. Dr. Jasper's scheme defines a set of

---

[2] http://www.aapb.org/news.html

electrode placements on the scalp whose relative position will be determined by the dimensions of each individual's head so that electrodes placed on heads of different dimensions will be in comparable locations on the scalp. This system is based on a set of latitudinal and longitudinal arcs upon the surface of an approximately spherical cranium, and positions of electrodes are determined by measurements from standard landmarks (i.e., nasion, inion, and preauricular points) on the skull. Arc length measurements from nasion to inion and from the preauricular point of one ear over vertex to the opposite ear are taken as well as a measurement around the circumference. Electrodes are then placed at locations 10, 20, 20, 20, 20, and 10% along each of these arcs.[3]

Jose Delgado

Jose Delgado, a professor of physiology at Yale University, is considered one of the world's most acclaimed and controversial neuroscientists. Delgado developed the brain chip, a device that could manipulate the brain by transmitting and receiving signals to and from neurons. Delgado implanted chips in the brains of animals and subsequently humans. He demonstrated that he could control certain behaviors through brain stimulation. His work was tested in patients who suffered from paralysis, epilepsy, blindness, Parkinson's disease, and other disorders.

Neal Miller and Leo DeCara

From Nealmiller.org:

> Neal Miller, Leo DeCara, and their colleagues carried out a series of dramatic animal experiments in the 1960s, demonstrating the operant conditioning of a variety of internal autonomically regulated physiologic processes, including blood pressure, cardiac function, and intestinal activity. Prior to their research, physiologists generally assumed that organisms have control over bodily functions governed by the central nervous system (or "voluntary nervous system"). The internal physiological processes controlled by the autonomic (or "involuntary") nervous system were regarded as operating beyond conscious awareness or control.
>
> Miller and DeCara used animals paralyzed by curare so that the animals could not produce the desired visceral changes through voluntary activity mediated by the central nervous system. In this paralyzed state their animal subjects were still able to change their visceral functions.
>
> Many of Neal Miller's experiments on curarized animals have not been successfully replicated, yet his animal studies spurred further investigations extending the same operant model of visceral learning to human subjects. More importantly, Miller's research inspired the hope that biofeedback can enable a human being to take a more active role in recovering and maintaining health. Further, it encouraged the dream

---

[3] http://www.patentstorm.us/patents/5518007/description.html

that human beings can aspire to previously unimagined levels of personal control over bodily states, reaching unprecedented states of wellness and self-control.[4]

Joe Kamiya: A Psychological Model

Joe Kamiya, a psychologist teaching at the University of Chicago, began experiments on brainwave frequencies in the 1960s utilizing a student population and basic medical grade EEG recording equipment. Kamiya attached a sensing electrode to the left occiput of a subject's head where alpha brainwaves are evident. Kamiya presented a tone to the subject, who was then asked to guess whether he or she was "in alpha." Kamiya was able to determine if the subject's guess was accurate through studying EEG readings. Kamiya went on to establish that people could control brainwaves that were previously thought to be involuntary states. Kamiya's findings resulted in the beginning of brainwave biofeedback.

Kamiya's original work reportedly was about anxiety, which is still an interesting topic to the psychology community; thus, Kamiya's work is characterized as a psychological approach. Kamiya's hypothesis was that increased amounts of alpha wave production could lead to decreases in state and trait anxiety. Kamiya's findings strongly supported his hypothesis. In considerable detail, he explored the best methods for training individuals in alpha wave production and its consequences. Unfortunately, not enough people in the field read and learn from his research; instead, they keep reinventing the wheel.

The field of NFB exploded after *Psychology Today* published an article in 1968 on Kamiya's work. The first meeting of biofeedback professionals occurred as part of the 1968 International Brain and Behavior Conference in Colorado. The following year the first specific meeting of biofeedback researchers was held in Santa Monica, California, with 142 people attending. At this meeting the attendees decided to name their group the Biofeedback Research Society—later changed to Biofeedback Society of America and then to the Association for Applied Psychophysiology and Biofeedback. In the 1970s and 1980s, biofeedback research languished. However, several professionals continued to push forward. Over the past decade, NFB and QEEG have flourished once again.

Maurice "Barry" Sterman

Barry Sterman, a professor emeritus in the departments of neurobiology and psychiatry at UCLA, is well known for his experiments on brainwave states in cats in 1965. Sterman accidentally discovered a specific EEG rhythm state while conducting operant conditioning experiments with cats. While waiting for a food reward, the cats produced the same brainwave pattern in the motor strip as when they were alert and motionless. Sterman named this spindling 13-19 Hz low-beta frequency EEG pattern "sensorimotor rhythm" (SMR).

In 1967 through serendipitous circumstances, Sterman found that his lab cats, which were trained in the previous unrelated SMR experiment to produce this frequency, increased their resistance to

---

[4] http://nealmiller.org

seizure when he exposed them to toxic chemicals that induced epileptic seizures. The results of Sterman's research were subsequently replicated with monkeys and humans.

The combined research of Sterman and others provided the basis for SMR/beta biofeedback training commonly used for ADHD, ADD, and attentional issues. Additionally, SMR/beta training was used for several years on patients with seizures when conventional medication therapies did not work. Subsequently, it was noted that children who were hyperactive experienced improvement in their seizure status, and also had improved behavior. In 1982, Sterman received a research grant from the National Institutes of Health (NIH) to further his research. In this study, the cats were exposed to hydrazine fuel—some cats had seizures, others did not. The cats that had experienced SMR training were more resistant to seizures. Sterman's work led to the discovery that scientists could study brainwaves and alter brainwave physiology.

Sterman decided to employ this same procedure on individuals with seizure disorders and learned that it reduced their incidence of seizures. Interestingly, he found that he could reverse the effects of this training and increase seizure frequency as well.

Joel Lubar

Joel Lubar, University of Tennessee, pioneered the use of neurofeedback on children with hyperactivity and without seizures in the 1970s. His major focus involved the use of EEG biofeedback for ADD/ADHD, depression, seizure disorders, Tourette Syndrome and related tic disorders, and certain specific learning disabilities. Joel and Judith Lubar developed a NFB protocol for treating ADHD by decreasing theta and increasing beta (classic landmarks for ADHD).

In 1995, Lubar's (Lubar et al, 1995) landmark study provided comparative pre- and post-treatment measurements of several parameters in over 100 individuals with ADHD who improved and in those who did not. The changes noted in the group receiving neurofeedback were nearly equivalent to changes reported for the medication group. Other completed studies have similar findings.

Today, Lubar continues to be one of the leaders in the use of NFB for attentional issues. He is pioneering and presenting a new type of training to locate current sources in the brain utilizing 19 electrodes and a new computerized mathematical technique called LORETA. It is expensive and complex, but he believes that it will allow practitioners to more precisely target neurofeedback training.

Margaret Ayers

Margaret Ayers's graduate training was in clinical neuropsychology. She used biofeedback therapy for different kinds of medical problems: drug addiction, alcoholism, head injury, stroke, cerebral palsy, and coma. Ayers noted that ADD is the result of anoxia,[5] stroke, birth trauma, or

---

[5] Anoxia: A total decrease in the level of oxygen, an extreme form of hypoxia or "low oxygen." The terms *anoxia* and *hypoxia* are used in various contexts. Hypoxia: a condition in which tissues

head injury. Until her death in March 2008, it was believed that Dr. Ayers performed more NFB sessions than any other individual in the field. She was responsible for the development of digital real-time neurofeedback equipment that sampled EEG at a rate that provided unparalleled definition of the raw EEG and filtered waveforms . Ayers was a master clinician without equal in her ability to interpret raw EEG patterns.

Barry Sterman and Joel Lubar: The Neuropsychological Arousal Model

At the same time that Sterman and Lubar were conducting their work, Margaret Ayers was a lab assistant working for Sterman. She was so impressed with their findings that she struck out on her own to develop equipment and protocols to train the general population. Sterman and Ayers focused on theta reduction rather than beta enhancement. Their approach to EEG training was characterized by Andrew Abarbanel as an arousal model.

Since Sterman and Lubar are neuropsychologists in the traditional research mold, this approach is referred as the neuropsychological arousal model. This model proposes that brainwave frequency changes globally in a fairly stereotypical pattern as a consequence of functions related to daily activities. As cognitive processing increases, alpha brainwaves decrease and beta, or desynchronized brainwaves, increase. As sensorimotor input to the brain decreases, SMR increases and attentiveness decreases. As vigilance decreases, theta waves increase.

Overall, this model appears to be fairly accurate even though exceptions occur. One such exception as observed by some researchers is that a midline theta rhythm in the 5 Hz range occurs briefly during a full memory search. More recent research has indicated another exception as theta's role in coordination of cortical activities. Other exceptions, too numerous to mention here, have been noted as well. It is a good idea to avoid being too rigid with regard to this perspective.

Niels Birbaumer

Niels Birbaumer, a German neuropsychologist whose experience dates back to the beginning of the field in the 1960s, is recognized for his pioneering work in slow cortical potential (SCP) EEG training, which included blind placebo-controlled studies applying the SCP NFB training to epilepsy. His more recent work at the National Institute of Health (NIH), focused on brain computer interface (BCI), evaluating many approaches to providing control over a computer, and thus a variety of prosthetic devices.

BCI involves acquiring brainwave signals that when amplified and input into a computer can be translated into messages or commands that reflect a person's intentions; it is a system that allows a person to communicate with or control the external world without involving the brain's normal output pathways.

---

are deprived of an adequate supply of oxygen. Apraxia is a neurological disorder characterized by loss of the ability to execute or carry out learned purposeful movements, despite having the desire and the physical ability to perform the movements.

Hershel Toomim

Dr. Hershel Toomim, a physicist, clinician, and researcher, is a pioneer in the field of psychophysiology and biofeedback and holds 22 patents for his inventions. He created the first biofeedback system to use telemetry, enabling patients to walk while disconnected from the central data collecting system. He developed one of the first publicly available neurofeedback units, known as the Alpha Pacer. In addition, Dr. Toomim developed hemoencephalography (HEG)—specifically, the study of voluntarily controlled blood flow, or oxygenation, to specifically chosen brain regions. He recently sold the patent on this technology. It should be available commercially in the near future. Not long ago, Toomim promoted the hypothesis that neurofeedback and HEG are effective because practitioners train the patient's brain (brainwaves) intentionally.

Elmer Green

From the Menninger Clinic:

> Elmer Green, Ph.D., researched and applied biofeedback techniques he developed in his ongoing study of "subtle energies," a field in which he remains preeminent. Dr. Green, the father of autogenic biofeedback training, was the first person ever to receive a National Institutes of Health (NIH) research grant, which was given for his autonomic research program (involuntary internal stimuli) at Menninger in the mid-1960s. The techniques he and his wife, Alyce Green, developed were used to train individuals how to achieve more control over their bodies in order to increase their physical and mental well-being.[6]

Green used biofeedback instruments to study Eastern yogis. He discovered that certain yogis could control their internal states merely through meditation and thought. His methods and techniques were adapted by Eugene Peniston and became what is now known as alpha-theta training. Dr. Soutar has expanded this approach into a method of neurofeedback known as deep states training.

Eugene Peniston

In the 1980s, Eugene Peniston at the VA Medical Center at Fort Lyon, Colorado, studied the effects of combining alpha-theta training with their existing program for alcoholics and published some of the first and most influential research about neurofeedback. Five years after participating in the program, 70% of the participants remained abstinent. Peniston researched alcoholism and theta activity. He noted that theta was lower in the back of the brain—often both theta and alpha were lower in the back of the brain. He and Paul Kulkosky continued to do groundbreaking research together at the Menniger Clinic on both alcoholism and post-traumatic stress disorder (PTSD). Peniston also consulted and guided Bill Scott on several pieces of research that attempted to replicate Peniston's findings.

---

[6] http://www.menningerclinic.com/about/Menninger-history.htm

Paul Kulkosky

The American Association of Experts in Traumatic Stress describes Kulkosky:

> Paul Kulkosky developed alpha training for alcoholism and PTSD. The Peniston/Kulkosky EEG alpha-theta neurofeedback protocol is being used by many practitioners to treat alcohol and other psychoactive substance disorders. Some alcohol treatment programs using the Peniston/Kulkosky EEG alpha-theta neurofeedback protocol as a primary treatment modality for alcohol addiction have demonstrated that intensive neurofeedback-based treatment has exerted a positive influence on a number of factors which contribute to alcohol intake including stress levels, depressive personality traits, beta endorphin output, resting levels of alpha and theta brainwaves, and prolonged abstinence. Data supporting the efficacy of the Peniston/Kulkosky method are of particular interest for the treatment of substance abuse because successful outcome is being discovered with patients who are difficult to treat in traditional alcohol treatment programs including patients with post-traumatic stress disorder and chronic alcoholic problems.[7]

Bill Scott

From Brain Paint:

> Bill Scott is the principal investigator and first author of an addiction research project that yielded a 79% success rate with Native American alcoholics. This study was with Dr. Eugene Peniston. An interview with Bill by the *Psychiatric Times* was published as a feature article. Bill Scott has also presented research at the American Association for the Advancement of Science with Dr. David Kaiser. Bill trained the researchers Dr. John Gruzelier and Dr. Tobias Egner (members of Department of Cognitive Neuroscience and Behaviour, Imperial College Medical School) in the use of alpha-theta protocols. The results of this research project so improved music abilities among Royal Conservatoiry of Music students that the Conservatoire has made these protocols a mandatory part of the school's curriculum.[8]

Elmer Green, Eugene Peniston, Nancy White, and Bill Scott: The Alpha-Theta Model

Elmer Green worked only briefly in the field, but left an indelible mark. With a background in biophysics, he experimented extensively with theta wave training—something that horrifies many practitioners today. Keep in mind that during that time, much of the emerging paradigm of biofeedback resulted from laboratory analysis of eastern yogis' abilities to control autonomic functions. He related the profound experiences that individuals had with works such as the yogic Aphorisms of Patanjali.

---

[7] http://www.aaets.org/arts/art47.htm
[8] http://www.brainpaint.com/index_files/aboutbillscott.htm

While Eugene Peniston was a managing psychologist at the Menninger Clinic, he enrolled in one of Green's workshops and was so impressed with the technology that he tried it with alcoholics. Paul Kulkosky, his associate, remarked that they noticed many alcoholics had a notable deficit of alpha. They thought that alpha training would help alcoholics while in recovery. When they consistently trained the alcoholics in alpha wave production over a period of several weeks, they found that it accelerated the alcoholics' recovery dramatically. Later they tried the same technique on PTSD patients with similar results. Their published studies were crucial contributions to establishing the early validity of neurofeedback as a psychological tool of considerable adjunctive value at the clinical level.

Nancy White is a past president of the International Society of Neurofeedback and Research (ISNR). She originally studied NFB with Adam Crane and began implementing and teaching it extensively. Her workshops inspired many clinicians to adapt the technique. As she worked with people over the years at the clinical level, she refined the technique and eventually developed a theoretical perspective that she detailed in her first textbook on the topic.

Bill Scott has achieved more for peer-reviewed research on alpha-theta training than just about anyone in the field of neurofeedback. His most recent research is a peer-reviewed controlled groups design completed in cooperation with the UCLA Department of Psychology. In it, Bill Scott and David Kaiser have combined both fast- and slow-wave training into a very effective, unique, and comprehensive approach. Unfortunately, few practitioners actually read Scott's research or take workshops to learn his techniques. Despite the amount of high-quality research, many practitioners have misconceptions about alpha-theta training; consequently, the approach is underutilized.

Alpha-theta is more attractive to practitioners who are clinically oriented and prefer to interact psycho-dynamically with their clients. It can be used for deep states training and tapping into client issues at a Jungian level. On the other hand, qualified practitioners such as Nancy White will often do no more than place the electrode on a client's head and still obtain good results. While success like hers is possible, a fair amount of coaching can assist the client greatly. Alpha-theta training has also been used effectively by many successful peak performance specialists such as Rae Tattenbaum.

Within the last 5-10 years, practitioners of neurofeedback have taken a second look at deep brain states. Alpha-theta training has been used in the treatment of alcoholism and other addictions, PTSD, the dysphoric disorders of women musicians, and psychopathic offenders. During this therapy, when the alpha wave amplitude is crossed over by the rising amplitude of theta waves, the state is called the alpha-theta crossover state and is associated with the resolution of traumatic memories. This low-frequency training differs greatly from the high-frequency beta and SMR training that has been practiced for over 30 years and is more reminiscent of the original alpha training of Elmer Green and Joe Kamiya.

Beta and SMR training can be considered a more direct physiological approach, strengthening sensorimotor inhibition in the cortex and inhibiting alpha patterns, which slows metabolism. On the other hand, alpha-theta training derives from the psychotherapeutic model and involves accessing of painful or repressed memories through the alpha-theta state.

The physiological mechanisms behind these therapies are currently unclear, but the theory is that repressed memories and unresolved traumas exert a stress on the brain that interferes with normal operation. EEGs of alcoholics reveal an inability to produce the alpha waves generally associated with feelings of relaxation and comfort. Theta and alpha waves increase after alcohol consumption. Since drowsiness and relaxation are common effects of alcohol, alcoholics may be self-medicating their abnormally low level of low frequency waves. Many studies demonstrate a high efficacy of alpha-theta therapy in treating alcoholism.

Jay Gunkelman

Jay Gunkleman is one of the most experienced clinical and research EEG/QEEG specialists in the world. He started in 1972 with the first state hospital-based biofeedback laboratory and has specialized in EEG for decades. He has authored many scientific papers and a mounting list of books. His depth of understanding of the mind/brain's function is unique. Jay is a popular lecturer world-wide and has occupied leadership positions in the field's professional societies.

Gunkelman runs a successful QEEG business. He tirelessly carries his equipment all over the world acquiring QEEGs and interpreting them for the neurofeedback community. His insights concerning the relationship between QEEG maps and neural functioning have helped professionals diagnose disorders and determine appropriate medications. Perhaps his most important contribution is his emerging method for determining the best protocols for neurofeedback intervention based on QEEG brain maps.

Robert W. Thatcher

Robert Thatcher is president and chief executive officer of Applied Neuroscience, Inc., a company that provides clinical report analysis, medical and legal evaluations, expert witnesses for court trials, research services, specialized analyses, specialized software pertaining to EEG, and quantitative analysis of the EEG. As president and CEO, Thatcher has both numerous and diverse responsibilities. His work is best noted for his research on head trauma (TBI), QEEG neurometrics, and Z-scores.

Applied Neuroscience, Inc., has developed a 19-channel instantaneous Z-score biofeedback program for purposes of neuroimage therapy or neuroimage biofeedback. Patients monitor their own brains in 3-D and in real-time to modify the electrical energies of their brains. Applied Neuroscience, Inc., also has developed a 2- and 4-channel dynamic link library, or DLL, based on the statistics of NeuroGuide for approved industry developers to use in their products. This DLL has provided real-time normative database comparisons for absolute power, power ratios, relative power, coherence, phase delays, and amplitude differences.

BrainMaster® is the first industry developer to incorporate the DLL into a complete biofeedback system. In addition, they have developed special techniques for advanced targeting methods and live feedback and they have published various technical reports and case studies using the new methods.

Thatcher spent a significant amount of time looking at TBI. He noted that at birth, infants' brainwaves are approximately 40% delta, but in adults these waves account for about 5%; thus elevated delta is often indicative of TBI. Kirtley Thornton and Dennis Carmody (2008) reported that QEEG identifies TBI approximately 90% of the time.

Thatcher did a great deal of research with head trauma and developed a database that has proven very accurate in diagnosing levels of severity. He also studied EEG and MRI together. This research provided new insights regarding the relationship between grey matter and white matter tissue damage and the resulting consequences in terms of EEG production in the brain. Much of his research focused on coherence. He produced important articles on this topic, which attracted considerable attention in the field of neurofeedback. Presently, Thatcher maintains one of the most widely used EEG databases in the field.

E. Roy John

Dr. E. Roy John was among the world's most recognized researchers in the fields of electrophysiology and biopsychology. He served as a research and development consultant with the Psychological Institute of Atlanta (PSI) and as a clinical consultant with QEEG and EP services offered through PSI. Dr. John and his wife, Leslie Prichep, performed all the initial research on the normative distribution of the human EEG and demonstrated that this distribution was consistent across culture, race, and gender. As a result, he developed the first neurometric database system and published research showing how EEG patterns correlate with various neuropsychological disorders. E. Roy John, in cooperation with the LEXICOR Corporation, supplied the first usable database for the neurofeedback community, NX Link, which provided a standard pattern of normative EEG.

Robert Thatcher and Jay Gunkelman: A QEEG Medical Perspective

Thatcher and Gunkleman probably have done more to promote quantitative EEG analysis (QEEG), or neurometrics, than anyone else in the field. Thatcher worked with E. Roy John developing EEG databases. He presented at the first ISNR meetings and conversed with neurofeedback providers and researchers. Gunkleman's original training was in the medical side of EEG. He immediately recognized the value of using databases for neurofeedback training. Gunkleman actively taught individuals in the neurofeedback community about the value, importance, and advantages of using QEEG.

QEEG involves collecting EEG signals from multiple sites on the scalp. These signals are then compared to a normative database to search for deviations from the mean values. These deviations are then usually reported in data tables and in the form of topographic maps. This process gives clinicians a fairly comprehensive picture of what is going on globally and locally in the brain in terms of EEG activity. This information can then be used to decide on an appropriate protocol for training.

Many clinicians like this approach because it provides a clear empirical basis for assessment and protocol decision making. It is also very well grounded in a wider research effort in the neuropsychology community. However, QEEG can be difficult to learn, and it has a longer learning curve than other approaches. It is very technical and often overwhelming to those who are used to more intuitive approaches. In addition, it requires very expensive equipment and databases. Therefore, not every professional is ready to dive into neurofeedback.

Although many professionals such as Marvin Sams proclaim that it is unethical to provide neurofeedback services without QEEG brain mapping, many others in the field have developed methods for protocol implementation that appear approximately if not equally as effective in results. At present there have not been enough replicated studies to confirm the superiority of one approach over the other. The clear value of QEEG is in assessment and tracking of abnormalities in the EEG.

Siegfried and Susan Othmer

This couple originally became involved in the field of neurofeedback to help their son. They produced some of the early reliable training equipment and developed a large network of affiliated practitioners who utilized their approach. Building primarily on the work of Sterman, they developed a basic and systematic approach to neurofeedback that does not use brain mapping and has proven very effective in dealing with a wide variety of disorders.

Siegfried's background in physics injected some very important challenging ideas into the field regarding research assumptions and theories about the relationship between neural functioning and EEG. At present, these concepts are very much under-appreciated. He is also one of the most outspoken commentators on the political and social implications of the work done in the field of neurofeedback.

Their early recognition of the role that asymmetry plays in proper neural functioning is particularly important. Much of their early technique involved balancing left and right hemispheres with respect to levels of arousal, or symptoms-based training.

In more recent times, Sue has shifted from monopolar training to an innovative bipolar training method that uses multiple sites across the scalp as well as sliding windows of uptraining and downtraining across the frequency spectrum. This new method is more symptom driven than past methods and results in rapid physiological responses to training. Client reports of changes in sensations, feelings, and symptoms often occur as soon as the session begins and protocols are changed accordingly. Sue has developed a very thorough taxonomy of symptoms and protocols that should be used in each case.

Many practitioners like this approach because it is very interactive and provides clear responses to each change. Others have complained that clients don't always know what they are feeling and don't report it effectively. This tendency makes protocol decisions very difficult. Some clinicians have expressed concerns that the protocols are so strong that they may be moving the clients too rapidly. However, it is overall one of the most popular and easy to learn approaches to neurofeedback.

Most recently, the Othmers have focused on low frequency training that involves the use of special electrodes and amplifiers designed for training below 1 Hz. Such training has been termed DC training, sub-delta training, or slow cortical potential training by various researchers and practitioners, and is hypothesized to affect shifting DC potentials that are the source of EEG activity.

Les Fehmi

Les Fehmi is director of the Princeton Biofeedback Centre and a founding member of the Biofeedback Society of America (now AAPB). For over thirty years, he conducted research and practiced clinically in the area of attention and EEG biofeedback. He developed Open Focus™ training and has specialized in multi-channel, alpha phase-synchrony neurofeedback, which he pioneered. His work is best understood by reading his book on Open Focus methods that he wrote in concert with Jim Robbins.

Adam Crane

Adam Crane is founder of the International MindFitness Foundation, which is dedicated to psychophysiological research and education, with a particular emphasis on developing and making available practical life and performance enhancement strategies and training programs. Since 1971, Crane and the organizations he founded or co-founded have provided leadership in the development of biofeedback hardware and software as well as innovative and effective business models for practitioners.

Les Fehmi and Adam Crane: The Profound Attention Model

Les Fehmi and Adam Crane have both focused on attention as a key to personal development and mental health. Their emphasis on attention is broader in scope than Joel Lubar's. Their approach also involves the metaphysical and the social-psychological. Both have focused on alpha training and synchrony as they relate to attention and influence mental functioning. Synchrony is a special form of brainwave coherence that is discussed later in the book. Fehmi has developed special equipment for training alpha synchrony, but it is not widely distributed at this point. He also has developed some very sophisticated techniques in attentional training.

Currently, he conducts workshops in these techniques that are experiential in nature and enlightening with regard to how much our perception and consciousness are regulated by our attention. The book *Mindfitness Training: Neurofeedback and the Process* includes Crane's perspective and a sample of his workshop called the Process (Crane & Soutar, 2000). Crane has also worked with others to develop specialized equipment for alpha training and synchrony training, but uses a definition of terms that is slightly different than that of Les Fehmi. In fact, Crane coined the term "profound attention," which he sees as the outcome of both alpha training and the process. He views this form of attentional development as antidotal to many of the modern dilemmas encountered, including mental disorder.

Peter Rosenfeld

Rosenfeld is best known for his depression protocol (1997) correcting the alpha asymmetry, a common finding with depression, noting that SMR can alter alpha asymmetry. Elsa Baehr collaborated with Rosenfeld to do research demonstrating the effectiveness of this technique for neurofeedback practitioners, which lead to its widespread clinical use.

Valdeane W. Brown

From Future Health:

> Dr. Valdeane W. Brown is an internationally recognized "trainer of trainers," who teaches and consults widely on personal and organizational transformation and computer systems. With a Ph.D. in clinical psychology and a background in math, physics, computer programming, philosophy, yoga, meditation, and martial arts, Dr. Brown brings a presence and precision to his work, informed by a deep sense of compassion, a profound facility with energy dynamics and commitment to revealing the elegant simplicity inherent in learning and transformation.[9]

Expanding on the work of others, Brown initially focused on training at C3 & C4. Brown is often misunderstood in the field because he deals in knowledge not understood by most practitioners: nonlinear dynamical theory and chaos theory. He has developed a technique and a computer program to implement this perspective. His approach involves training both sides of the brain at the same time using multiple frequencies and reinforcement tones. He has provided regular workshops on the topic.

Period 3 techniques have three basic stages and training frequencies are altered at each stage. Some practitioners have doubted the ability of clients to hear and respond to so much feedback activity, but his clients appear to do quite well. Brown maintains that his outcomes are just as good as those who use brain maps, if not better. More recently, Brown has utilized his NeuroCare Pro system to generate a more seamless and automated neurofeedback approach that he has marketed to individuals and practitioners. He feels that his expert system is sophisticated enough that even home users can hook themselves up and effectively train without the guidance of a professional practitioner.

Anna Wise: The High Performance Mind

Anna does not use EEG biofeedback in the same way that others in the field typically use it. She originally worked with Maxwell Cade, who traveled the world measuring the EEG of reportedly enlightened individuals and other peak performers. Her program is the result of his findings and her insights into his work. Rather than employ operant conditioning directly, she has created mental exercises to develop the mind and evaluate progress using specially designed EEG equipment. Her method of "neuromonitoring," as she refers to it, allows her to work with groups of individuals to access an "awakened mind" state providing profound breakthroughs and insights.

Anna's workshops have attracted those interested in deep states training as well as groups working toward insight and spiritual growth. Due to recent problems with her health, Anna has

---

[9] http://www.futurehealth.org/populum/authors_productpage.php?sid=418

not been able to do her workshops as often as in the past. In fact, there is some concern within the community that her approach may not survive. Fortunately, a few individuals are trying to incorporate her approach into their own styles and present similar workshops. Her books, *The High Performance Mind* and *The Awakening Mind,* are very well written and provide the best introduction to her work. Both are excellent sources for practitioners.

KEY TRAINERS IN THE FIELD OF NEUROFEEDBACK

Michael and Lynda Thompson

Michael and Lynda Thompson are pioneers in the field of neurofeedback in Canada. They are strong advocates of integrating biofeedback with neurofeedback together in the clinical setting and have led the field in this area, presenting some of the best techniques for utilizing both paradigms. Much of their initial focus was on ADD. They have worked closely with Thought Technology and developed many of their innovative techniques and protocols around Thought Technology equipment. They have published an excellent book on neurofeedback entitled *The Neurofeedback Book*. Over the years they have conducted hundreds of workshops and played a key role in training other practitioners.

Jon Anderson

Jon Anderson has worked with biofeedback and neurofeedback since 1974 and has been one of the key neurofeedback trainers. As a clinician, he has experimented extensively with all of the innovations in the field. He has worked closely with the Stens Corporation and has earned the reputation of being one of the best and most informed instructors available.

Len Ochs

From Future Health: "Len Ochs is a psychologist in private practice, working in biofeedback since 1975 and psychotherapy since 1966. He is considered one of the pioneers in biofeedback—especially in the area of instrumentation development."[10] Len Ochs is most recognized for the development of The Low Energy Neurofeedback System (LENS), which was registered by the FDA in April, 2009.

LENS uses a device, under control of a computer program, to produce electromagnetic fields and apply them as brain stimuli. The stimuli are applied by EEG leads that serve as bi-directional conduits for both the stimuli and returning EEG signals. Treatment sessions are very short, typically only a few minutes. Treatments that are too long or use incorrect settings can cause hyper-arousal, headache, irritability, nausea, etc. During treatment sessions, the subject is completely passive; there is no auditory or visual feedback.

LENS treatment is preceded by a diagnostic QEEG brain map to identify zones of the brain where various brainwaves deviate from the norm. Both electrode placement and system settings are determined by the condition being treated and the clinician's interpretation of the brain map.

---

[10] http://www.futurehealth.org/populum/authors_productpage.php?sid=424

System settings must be adjusted by the clinician over the course of treatment to accommodate the effects of treatment. The number of treatments needed to improve ADD/ADHD, depression, PTSD, and seizures is claimed to be fewer than for more traditional neural feedback methods.

Richard Soutar

Richard pioneered clinical work with entrainment and QEEG database systems. He co-developed a hand-held neurofeedback trainer with Dave Siever and collaborated with BrainMaster developing new concepts models for clinical implementation, such as home training and the MiniQ. He is best known for his innovative work in deep states training and neuromeditation—the use of neurofeedback to assist in achieving altered states and meditation. Recently, he developed an internet-based Expert Database System for comprehensive clinical use that involves assessment measures along a bio-psycho-social model. It assesses social behavior, cognitive behavior, and physiological symptoms and correlates them with QEEG analysis to rapidly generate a clinically friendly report. This system is a critical step to making QEEG more accessible to clinicians of all types and enhances the visibility of the discipline.

SUMMARY

All of these practitioners were in the field before brain mapping was available. They and major research facilities developed methods without that important resource. Despite the lower price of brain mapping equipment and databases, many of these practitioners still do not rely on brain maps and are quite successful in their practices. While still recognizing the validity of other approaches, the ISNR recently published a paper recommending the use of QEEG brain mapping for assessment purposes. This perspective becomes more understandable by viewing QEEG primarily as an assessment and tracking tool and not the sole basis for protocol determination.

None of the mentioned perspectives is exclusive in the interpretation of neurofeedback. In fact, there is considerable overlap among them. This book weaves these perspectives together, so that the underlying relationships become more obvious.

As they do in most fields, politics surround these perspectives. Also, many technological advancements have been developed for use with these perspectives. However, interesting equipment and programs may or may not work with a specific perspective. Consequently, many practitioners entering the field find themselves purchasing several different pieces of equipment in order to use several perspectives clinically. Others become locked into one expensive piece of equipment and perspective without the ability to change.

Not all perspectives reflect the mainstream research. Learning one type of terminology unique to a cutting-edge perspective can limit dialogue with other practitioners and more mainstream research. In the long run, practitioners are likely to be served best by investigating several different approaches and developing their own "tool boxes."

The Appendices at the end of this book contain a list of leading companies and training programs for those interested.

Review Questions

1) What series of dramatic animal experiments did Neal Miller and DeCara conduct in the 1960s?

2) Barry Sterman is most known for his work with what experiments?

3) Joe Kamiya is recognized for what contribution to biofeedback?

4) Joel Lubar's major focus of work involves the use of EEG biofeedback for treating what disorder?

5) What did Herbert Jasper develop?

6) What did Hans Berger discover?

7) Eugene Peniston is best known for his work using neurofeedback to treat what population?

8) What was Richard Canton the first to discover?

9) Is neurofeedback considered to be experimental?

CHAPTER 2: ANATOMY, ELECTROPHYSIOLOGY AND THE BRAIN

To understand EEG and its origin, it is best to begin with a study of the basic anatomy and neurophysiology of the brain. Becoming proficient with terms and concepts relating to this topic will make reading the scientific literature easier and contribute significantly to the ability to provide effective neurofeedback protocols.

BRAIN DEVELOPMENT AND STRUCTURES

The human brain goes through a complex process of development starting at birth and continuing through adolescence into adulthood. Even in later adult years, the brain remains plastic and new brain cells are created. The brain develops from bottom to top, right to left, and back to front. It has many structures, regions, and parts, including the cerebral cortex, brain stem, cerebellum, four lobes, two hemispheres, and limbic system. It is vital to know and understand these structures to use EEG and NFB.

THE NEOCORTEX AND CORTEX

Vertically, the brain (also referred to as the triune brain) can be divided into three parts: the brain stem, the limbic system, and the neocortex. The triune brain recognizes that the three major regions of the brain evolved over time, creating separate but interdependent systems: the brain stem and cerebellum (reptilian brain), the emotional brain (limbic system or mammalian brain), and the thinking brain (the cortex).

From a horizontal perspective, the brain can be divided into two parts: the right and left cerebral hemispheres.

P. T. Stien and J. Kendall note that the neocortex are responsible for both cognition and metacognition—the ability to think about thoughts, emotions, and behavior (2004). The neocortex is responsible for the "executive functioning" of the person. It determines personality, goals, and decisions, and guides the following:

- reasoning
- weighing choices
- concrete and abstract thought
- inductive and deductive reasoning
- cause-and-effect relationships
- delaying actions
- planning

- goal-directed behavior

The neocortex controls cognitive memory that includes facts, figures, faces, names, and dates.

The cortex has six layers. The white matter underneath contains the wiring that connects the cortex for long-distance communication.

INDIVIDUAL BRAIN CELLS LIVE IN "COLUMNS." USING AN OFFICE ANALOGY:

- The top layers are similar to inter-office memos.
- The middle layers are like the "inbox."
- The bottom layers serve as the "outbox."

Most of the EEG we capture from the scalp is from the top layers. The term used for these EEG-producing areas is "dipole layer." The EEG they produce does not register at the scalp until neurons over an area of about at least 6 cm resonate together.

The neuron (individual brain cell) is the cell body that receives information from other cells connected to its dendrites. The other cells' signals vote on whether this cell should fire a signal. The cell body develops an electrical charge or signal in response to the votes, and then the signal travels down the axon to other cells to vote as well. The waxing and waning of these "voting charges" from layers two and three of the cortex come together to create the EEG.

Neurons live in adjacent cell columns that permeate the cortex layers. Axons spread between adjacent cell columns to create "local" connections (beta-gamma resonances). Axons travel somewhat longer distances to generate regional connections (alpha to beta resonances). Axons travel long distances to generate global connections (delta to theta resonances).

In the cortex, information flows over several major channels or nerve bundles called fasciculae. Information traveling between left and right hemispheres goes through the corpus callosum and anterior commissure. While front to back information travels through the cingulum, uncinate, and arcurate fasciculae, the two major flow zones meet in the frontal region. Convergence zones (such as the posterior temporal region) are major interface zones.

Recently, it has been discovered that the brain is organized around major "hubs" that help coordinate brain network activity (Hagmann et al., 2008). The majority of these hubs are in the parietal region, the ventromedial frontal region, and the temporal lobes. These hubs are so critical to effective functioning that damage to any one of them results in extensive impairment of whole regions of brain networks. Conversely, damage outside these hub areas remains relatively contained to local areas.

ORIENTATION TO THE BRAIN

THE CEREBRUM (BETA)

The cerebrum or cortex (cerebral cortex) is the largest part of the human brain, making up 80% of the brain's mass, and is a six-layered structure that performs different functions. The cerebral cortex is the gray matter that covers the outermost layer of the brain like the bark of a tree and generates beta wave activity. Beneath it is all the white matter that constitutes the wiring between the different areas of the cortex. Subcortical systems include the following:

- limbic system or midbrain (emotion and memory)
- brain stem or hindbrain (survival functions)
- cerebellum (coordinates timing, fine movement, balance, motor sequencing)
- pineal gland (an endocrine gland that produces the hormone melatonin)
- thalamus (sensory and motor functio0ns)
- hypothalamus (regulates sexual drive, thirst, hunger)
- pituitary gland (controls all the other glands)

Nerve cells make up the gray surface of the cerebrum, which is a little thicker than a thumb. White nerve fibers, underneath, carry signals between the nerve cells and other parts of the brain and body.

The cortex is the thinking part of the brain, responsible for people's ability to plan, reason, and consciously "think" about what they do. In other words, the human urges and emotions generated by the limbic system pass through neurological pathways to the cortex, where they are processed. In general, the function of the cortex is higher-level information processing. When it is engaged in this processing, it tends to generate more beta waves.

The cortex has to make sense of and figure out how to respond to and satisfy these urges. This is the most sophisticated part of the brain and can be described from a structural-functional perspective by dividing it into regions or lobes according to their specialization. These lobes are demarcated by fissures, or sulci. For instance, the back (posterior) section of the cortex is devoted mostly to vision and is called the occipital cortex. The prefrontal cortex (anterior) performs executive functions related to decision making. The temporal lobes (lateral) of the cortex are involved in memory, emotional processing and hearing. The cerebral cortex is highly wrinkled. Essentially, this feature makes the brain more efficient because it can increase the surface area of the brain and the amount of neurons within it (cortical folding). A deep furrow divides the cerebrum into two halves, the left and right hemispheres, with each side functioning slightly differently.

The prefrontal cortex, at the front tip of the brain, is the socio-emotional supervisor. It is the part of the brain that helps people stay focused, make plans, control impulses, and make good (or bad) decisions.

The cingulate, a part of the brain that runs longitudinally underneath and through the middle of the frontal lobes, is the "gear shifter." It allows people to shift attention from thought to thought and between behaviors.

The cerebral cortex is divided into four sections called "lobes": the frontal lobes, temporal lobes, parietal lobes, and occipital lobes.

Knowledge of the brain and its functioning continues to expand almost daily. Current research supports much of what has been learned about the brain and its functions through QEEG brain mapping and work with neurofeedback. The following excerpt from *Science Daily* is an example:

Neuroscientists Map Intelligence in the Brain

Neuroscientists at the California Institute of Technology (Caltech) have conducted the most comprehensive brain mapping to date of the cognitive abilities measured by the Wechsler Adult Intelligence Scale (WAIS), the most widely used intelligence test in the world. The results offer new insight into how the various factors that comprise an "intelligence quotient" (IQ) score depend on particular regions of the brain.

Neuroscientist Ralph Adolphs, professor of psychology and neuroscience, and professor of biology at Caltech, Caltech postdoctoral scholar Jan Gläscher, and their colleagues compiled the maps using detailed magnetic resonance imaging (MRI) and computerized tomography (CT) brain scans of 241 neurological patients recruited from the University of Iowa's extensive brain-lesion registry.

All of the patients had some degree of cognitive impairment from events such as strokes, tumor resection, and traumatic brain injury, as assessed by testing using the WAIS. The WAIS test is composed of four indices of intelligence, each consisting of several subtests, which together produce a full-scale IQ score. The four indices are the verbal comprehension index, which represents the ability to understand and produce speech and use language; the perceptual organization index, which involves visual and spatial processing, such as the ability to perceive complex figures; the working memory index, which represents the ability to hold information temporarily in mind (similar to short-term memory); and the processing speed index.

The authors correlated the four major domains of intelligence (verbal comprehension, perceptual organization, working memory and processing speed, represented by the pictograms) with the lesion maps of over 240 patients. The findings provide the first voxelwise mapping of where in the brain focal damage can compromise intelligence factors.

Somewhat surprisingly, the study revealed a large amount of overlap in the brain regions responsible for verbal comprehension and working memory, which suggests that these two now-separate measures of cognitive ability may actually represent the same type of intelligence, at least as assessed using the WAIS.

The details about the structure of intelligence provided by the study could be useful in future revisions of the WAIS test so that its various subtests are grouped on the basis of neuroanatomical similarity rather than on behavior, as is the case now.

In addition, the brain maps produced by the study could be used as a diagnostic aid. Clinicians could combine the maps with their patients' Wechsler test results to help localize likely areas of brain damage. "It wouldn't be sufficient to be diagnostic, but it would provide information that clinicians could definitely use about what parts of the brain are dysfunctional," Adolphs says. (Gläscher et al., 2009)

THE LOBES OF THE BRAIN

FRONTAL LOBES

The frontal lobes (see Diagram 1: Lobes of the Brain, page 23) are the most anterior part of the cortex. They are located right under the forehead, and are responsible for the following:

- consciousness
- how people know what they are doing within their environment
- executive function
- attention
- motivation
- thinking
- problem solving
- judgments
- planning
- how people initiate activity in response to their environment
- movement and motor execution
- memory
  - o   short-term memory
  - o   memory for habits and motor activities
- emotions (current evidence indicates that emotion may be lateralized to both hemispheres)
  - o   mood control
  - o   emotional response or inhibition
  - o   emotional valancing
- language
  - o   expressive language
  - o   parts of speech
  - o   word associations
  - o   assigns meaning to the words we choose

The frontal lobes have three primary network systems (Chow & Cummings, 1998):

1) The orbital frontal network for processing socio-emotional information

2) The anterior cingulate network for processing attentional information

3) The dorsolateral network for processing memory

They bring together and coordinate information from the limbic system, the posterior processing areas, and temporal lobes. These are important key networks to test and evaluate in clients as they contribute significantly to social and academic performance.

The right frontal lobe controls emotion and expression of language or prosody.[11] Problems occurring there can lead to social problems, poor peer relations, and problems with authority. Children with problems in this area may be diagnosed with oppositional defiance disorder or conduct disorder. Elation can also occur when there is damage to or problems with the right frontal lobe. Conversely, depression occurs when damage or problems occur to the left frontal lobe.

Diagram 1: Lobes of the Brain

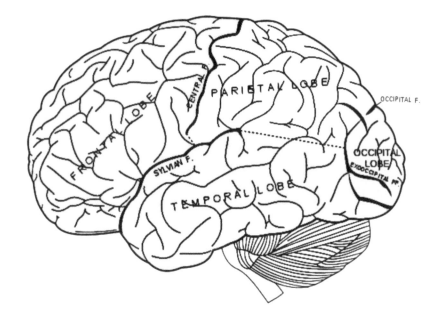

---

[11]Prosody is the rhythm, stress, and intonation of speech, and may reflect the emotional state of a speaker.

PARIETAL LOBES

The parietal lobes (see Diagram 1: Lobes of the Brain, above) are located near the back and top of the head. They are responsible for math and grammar; association between self, the environment, and others; and sensorimotor perception, integration of visual, and somatospatial information.

The parietal lobes are associated with the following:

- movement
    - goal-directed voluntary movements
    - manipulation of objects
- body awareness
    - arousal
    - perception of stimuli
- orientation (location)
    - location for visual attention
    - location for touch perception
- the integration of different senses that allows for understanding a single concept
- recognition
- association
- naming objects

The left parietal lobe governs language, math, and meaning construction, and can reflect language difficulties. The right parietal lobe governs arousal, facial decoding, and receptive prosody. People with Asperger's syndrome often demonstrate a lack of social integration, poor perception of others, and poor perception of self in relationship to others.

The angular gyrus is in the left parietal lobe that lies near the superior edge of the temporal lobe and immediately posterior to the supramarginal gyrus. It is Brodmann area 39 of the human brain (see Diagram 7: Brodmann Areas, page 36) and involved in a number of processes related to language, cognition, reading comprehension, and meaning construction.

TEMPORAL LOBES

The temporal lobes (see Diagram 1: Lobes of the Brain, page 23) are located on the sides of the head above the ears, underneath the temples, and behind the eyes. They are connected to the hippocampus, and are involved with the following:

- memory acquisition
    - short-term and long-term memory
- emotional valencing
    - temper control and aggression
- understanding language
    - comprehension
    - language function
- perception

- recognition of auditory stimuli and auditory perception
- some visual perceptions
- facial recognition
- categorization of objects and color

The temporal lobes are a major convergence zone. The left temporal lobe governs differentiation in language, receptive language, and auditory processing. When there are problems, especially in the left temporal lobe, people are more prone to temper flare-ups, rapid mood shifts, and memory and learning problems. Dyslexia results from damage to the temporal, parietal, or occipital lobes.

OCCIPITAL LOBES

The occipital lobes (see 1, above) are the smallest of the four true lobes in the human brain. They are located in the rearmost portion of the skull and are associated with visual processing, sequential memory functions, and arousal. In addition, they have connections with the cerebellum that involve the visual vestibular system, which affects balance and the amygdala. The occipital lobes contain most of the anatomical region of the visual cortex.

Diagram 2: Cross Section of the Brain

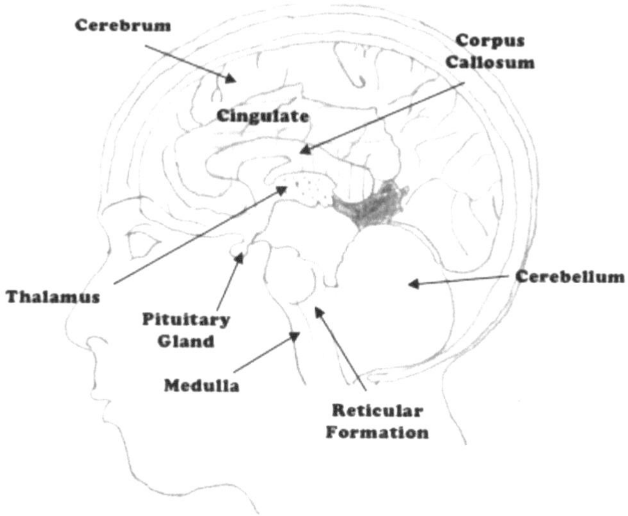

RIGHT AND LEFT HEMISPHERES

The right and left hemispheres are connected by the corpus callosum (a band of approximately three hundred million nerve cell fibers, which allows conscious information to be exchanged between hemispheres). It is larger in women than in men and has been identified as critically correlated with emotional intelligence. When children have been severely abused, the corpus callosum is often damaged and smaller than normal as a result. In gifted people, the corpus callosum is often larger than average (Terry Anderson, personal communication). The anterior commissure is another pathway that lies beneath the corpus callosum. It carries unconscious, emotional information between the two hemispheres and is a key pathway for emerging emotional feelings. Each hemisphere of the brain is dominant for certain functions and behaviors. In normal people, the two hemispheres are connected, work together, and share information through the corpus callosum.

The right hemisphere is slightly larger in normal adults, and is responsible for the following:

- Emotional quotient (E.Q.)
- swearing
- early self-concept
- social encoding
- social skills
- face recognition
- emotional processes
  - negative emotions
  - empathy
- nonverbal expression and association
- spatial memory and problem solving
- auditory processing
- musical processing

The left hemisphere is generally responsible for the following:

- I.Q.
- logic
- verbal association
- verbal expression
- verbal memory
- auditory processing
- word recognition
- math and grammar problem solving

Left-side brain problems often correspond with a tendency toward significant irritability and even violence.

THE BRAIN STEM AND CEREBELLUM (DELTA)

The brain stem connects the limbic system and the thalamus to the spinal cord and helps regulate the basic life functions of the body, such as heart rate, blood pressure, body temperature, respiration, consciousness, and primary states of arousal ranging from sleep to hyper-vigilance. It also controls the production and release of some neurotransmitters. Neurotransmitter abnormalities are associated with psychiatric disorders such as depression and psychosis (Ziegler, 2002). During deep sleep, the brain stem generates simple delta waves and resonates with cortical generators. The brain stem is the first part of the brain to develop before birth, and brain stem cells are generated directly from the human heart.

The cerebellum (see Diagram 3: The Brain, page 28) is located just above the brain stem and controls coordination and motor performance as well as social, emotional, and cognitive functions. The cerebellum accounts for 40% of neurological connections. It coordinates the timing of the entire brain and remembers all the motor sequences for learned behavior. The brain stem is made of the midbrain, pons, and medulla. The midbrain is involved in functions such as vision, hearing, eye movement and body movement.

The anterior part has the cerebral peduncle, which is a huge bundle of axons traveling from the cerebral cortex through the brain stem. These fibers (along with other structures) are important for voluntary motor function.

The pons (see Diagram 3: The Brain, page 28) is involved in motor control and sensory analysis. For example, information from the ear first enters the brain in the pons. It is important for regulating levels of consciousness and for sleep. Some structures within the pons are linked to the cerebellum and are involved in movement and posture.

The medulla oblongata is the caudal-most (posterior) part of the brain stem, between the pons and spinal cord. It is responsible for maintaining vital body functions, such as breathing and heart rate.

The cerebellum (Diagram 3: The Brain, page 28) is attached to the stem at the back and is involved in maintaining subroutines of the finer aspects of movement, such as dancing, writing, or playing a musical passage. The reticular activation system (RAS) also resides here and has a great deal to do with modulating levels of arousal. Antonio Demasio (1994) believes that consciousness itself emerges in this area of the stem above the area where the trigeminal nerve enters. The reticular formation greatly impacts the power of the EEG at any given time. The RAS and hypothalamus have very dense interconnections controlling many of the basic bodily functions and hormonal functions via the pituitary gland. Irregularities in these functions may be manifest in delta wave abnormalities.

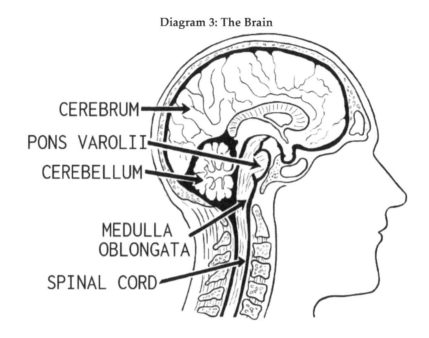

Diagram 3: The Brain

CEREBRUM

PONS VAROLII

CEREBELLUM

MEDULLA
OBLONGATA

SPINAL CORD

BASAL GANGLIA

The basal ganglia (see Diagram 4: Striatum or Basal Ganglia, page 29) are large structures deep within the brain. They control the body's idling speed (anxiety level). The basal ganglia integrate feelings, thoughts, and movement, and help to shift and smooth motor behavior. They allow for smooth integration of emotions, thoughts, and physical movement. When the basal ganglia are overactive, people are more likely to be overwhelmed by stressful situations. They may experience anxiety, panic, increased awareness, conflict avoidance, or heightened fear. Often they have a tendency to freeze or become immobile in thoughts or actions. These people are at risk for increased muscle tone or tremors that may result in headaches.

Underactive basal ganglia can cause problems with motivation, energy, and get-up-and-go. In addition, increased basal ganglia activity is often associated with anxiety that in turn can intensify pain. Increased left-sided basal ganglia activity is often seen in people who are chronically irritable or angry.

People with basal ganglia problems are often experts at predicting the worst (have negative outlook) and have an abundance of negative thoughts. It is interesting that thoughts affect every cell in the body. In fact, the constant stress from negative predictions lowers immune system effectiveness and increases the risk of becoming ill.

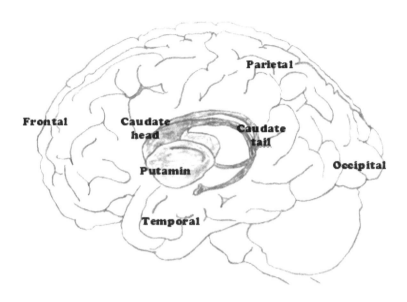

THE LIMBIC SYSTEM (THETA)

The cingulate is beneath the outer covering of the cortex, followed by the corpus callosum, and then a collection of smaller structures called the limbic structures. These structures surround the thalamus. The limbic system, which forms a ring around the brain stem, is dedicated to survival and is composed of the thalamus, hypothalamus, amygdala, hippocampus, basal ganglia, cingulate cortex, and septum.

The diencephalons include the thalamus and hypothalamus that mediate arousal, appetite, sex drive, autonomic arousal, muscle tone, and bracing. James Papez, a researcher in the first half of the twentieth century, first identified the limbic system as involved with processing emotional information and memory. The primary frequency generated by the limbic system is theta. It appears to emanate especially from a group of structures that make up a circuit at the heart of the system involving the septum and the hippocampus.

The limbic system (see Diagram 5, below), often referred to as the "emotional brain," is found buried within the cerebrum. From an evolutionary perspective, it is rather old. The limbic system controls autonomic functions with its direct connection to the hypothalamus and is also connected to the cortical and subcortical regions of the brain[12] through the right orbitofrontal

---

[12] Subcortical systems of the brain include the brain stem (survival functions) and cerebellum (coordinates fine movement).

area, which in turn regulates arousal, emotions, and behavior (the socio-emotional part of the brain).

Diagram 5: Limbic System

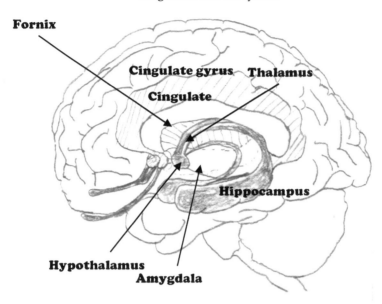

The limbic system in part regulates and affects perception, experience, and memory. It can be directly affected by psychological trauma. The amygdala is important in memory and has connections to all areas involved with emotions; the hippocampus stores short-term memory. The cingulate gyrus is a neocortical structure with 6 layers. The thalamus organizes and synchronizes the brain and, like the cingulate, is a key gatekeeper for all incoming sensory information.

The limbic system, especially the hypothalamus, controls the sleep and appetite cycles of the body. The hypothalamus is responsible for translating emotional states into physical feelings, relaxation, or tension. The front half of the hypothalamus sends calming signals to the body through the parasympathetic nervous system. The back half of the hypothalamus sends stimulating or fear signals to the body through the sympathetic nervous system. The back half is responsible for the fight-or-flight response. When the limbic system is "turned on," emotions tend to take over. When it is cooled down, more activation is possible in the cortex. Current research shows a correlation between depression, increased limbic system activity and shutdown in the prefrontal cortex—especially on the left side.

The limbic system and the temporal lobes store highly charged emotions and memories, both positive and negative. Cyclic mood disorders often correlate with focal areas of increased activity in the limbic system specifically and a patchy uptake across the surface of the brain in general. Limbic problems often correlate with cyclical tendencies toward depression and irritability. The importance of understanding the limbic system will be more apparent in the next chapter on EEG.

THE THALAMUS (ALPHA)

The thalamus (Diagram 5, page 30) is a walnut-sized structure at the center of each hemisphere. It acts as the relay station for incoming sensory stimuli and permits the senses to be used in combination. The structure has sensory and motor functions. All sensory information coming into the body goes through the thalamus, which is divided up into regions that correspond to different areas of the brain. The sensory information enters this structure where neurons send that information to the overlying cortex. Axons from every sensory system (except olfaction) synapse here as the last relay site before the information reaches the cerebral cortex.

The thalamus has multiple functions. As one thalamic projection may reach one or several regions in the cortex, it is believed to both process and relay sensory information selectively to various parts of the cerebral cortex. The thalamus plays a significant role in regulating arousal, the level of awareness, and activity. It is also responsible for regulating sleep states and wakefulness. Damage to the thalamus can lead to permanent coma, as well as pervasive memory loss.

The thalamus is thought of as the pacemaker of the brain, and its dominant rhythm appears to be alpha. Research suggests that the thalamus may engage and disengage different areas of the cortex through a resonance process involving the use of alpha as a form of braking. Research done by Sterman and Bowersox (1981) also shows that it clearly employs one frequency, SMR, in a gating system to control information flowing to and from a section of the cortex that controls primary motor functions.

HYPOTHALAMUS

The hypothalamus (Diagram 5, page 30) is a pea-sized structure that lies below the thalamus just above the brain stem and is responsible for certain metabolic processes as well as other activities of the autonomic nervous system (ANS). It synthesizes and secretes neurohormones, often called hypothalamic-releasing hormones. These in turn stimulate or inhibit the secretion of pituitary hormones. It works to maintain homeostasis and is the main center for information exchange between the brain and body, such as the following:

- control of the autonomic nervous system blood pressure
- circadian rhythms and cycles[13]
- emotion
    - i.e. anger and aggressive behavior
- thirst
- hunger
- fatigue
- body temperature
- glucose level

---

[13] A circadian rhythm is an approximate daily 24-hour cycle in the biochemical, physiological, or behavioral processes of living beings.

The hypothalamus links the nervous system to the endocrine system via the pituitary gland and has extensive links to the brain stem. The amygdala has overriding control in periods of high stress.

AMYGDALA

The amygdala (Diagram 5, page 30) is an almond-shaped structure located just beneath the surface of the front, medial part of the temporal lobe. It causes the bulge on the surface called the uncus. It is involved in memory, emotion, and fear. The amygdala is a component of the limbic system that stores memories of fearful experiences (traumatic memories). It monitors incoming stimuli for anything threatening and activates the fight-flight-freeze stress response when danger is detected. The amygdala is responsible for precipitating changes in heart rate, and blood pressure in response to threats. It works via the hypothalamus, brain stem, and the parasympathetic and sympathetic nervous systems. The amygdala stimulates production of brainwave patterns in the basal part of the frontal lobes (prefrontal cortex). The frontal lobe is one of the few structures that can effectively inhibit the amygdala through activation, which appears as increased beta.

HIPPOCAMPUS

The hippocampus (Diagram 5, page 30) is a finger-sized cluster of neurons located in the cerebral hemispheres in the basal medial part of the temporal lobe. Like a memory chip in a computer, the hippocampus is the hub of memory and learning. All conscious memory must be processed through the hippocampus. It is also important for converting short-term memory to more permanent long-term memory and for recalling spatial relationships.

The hippocampus is involved with verbal and emotional memory and is vulnerable to traumatic stress. With stress, the hippocampus shuts down the immune system and the IGA level goes down, which is related to fear. The hippocampus and particularly the amygdala provide conditioned learning and the ability to learn by association.

REVIEW QUESTIONS

4) What areas of the brain generate the four major brainwaves?

5) Name 3 functions of the frontal lobes.

6) Memories are stored in what area(s) of the brain?

7) What is the triune brain?

8) The brain stem is responsible for what function(s)?

CHAPTER 3: WHAT IS EEG?

THE BRAIN AND CLINICAL THEORY

Neurometrics is the quantitative EEG of the brain. The most practical way to consider the brain in relation to clinical theories and applications is to look at it in terms of cortical and subcortical processes (see Chapter 2 for further discussion about brain anatomy and neurophysioology). From an evolutionary perspective the subcortical structures are older and appear to have a greater overall influence on how the organism conducts its day-to-day business. The cortex, however, is the structure that is most associated with functions considered especially human. These two structures appear to work together, to some extent in parallel harmony. When disorders emerge, it is this relationship that is most disturbed.

The goal of this chapter is first to review the basic important anatomical features for those who are less familiar with this topic, and then to explore in deeper detail their structure, function, and the interrelationship of these features as these apply to neurotherapy protocols.

THE SOMATOSENSORY CORTEX/SENSORY MOTOR RHYTHM (SMR)

The somatosensory cortex (SMC) is part of two strips of tissue that are dedicated to sensory information and to motor functions (see Diagram 6: Motor and Somatosensory Cortex, page 35). The SMC runs bilaterally aross the cortex from ear to ear. Areas of each strip are specifically dedicated to corresponding areas of the body where the information originates and to which it flows back. Information flowing to and from these areas can be controlled through a gating system in the thalamus that opens and closes when a specific frequency, SMR, is generated by local thalamic cells.

THE SPLIT BRAIN

All information coming from the right hemisphere is related to the left side of the body and vice versa. The visual field is divided into two sections, left and right, in each eye. Each left side of each eye goes to the right brain and each right side of each eye goes to the left brain. Although these pathways are not 100% exclusive, they are fairly dedicated. This is important to know when employing entrainment devices to stimulate the left or right hemisphere at specific frequencies.

Diagram 6: Motor and Somatosensory Cortex[14]

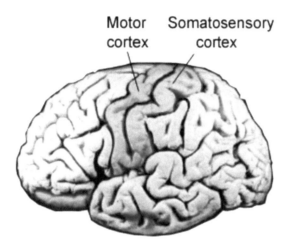

Motor cortex   Somatosensory cortex

THE BRODMANN AREAS

The structure of the brain can further be differentiated based on types of cells found in the brain that cluster together in areas or regions. Korbinian Brodmann, a German neurologist who is famous for his system of dividing the cerebral cortex into 52 distinct regions based upon their cyto-architectonic (histological) characteristics. He created a map that shows these regions, which are relatively stable across species of mammals. These areas are now usually referred to as Brodmann areas (Diagram 7: Brodmann Areas, page 36. A Brodmann area is a region of the cortex that is defined based on its organization of cells. Some of these areas were later associated to nervous functions, such as areas 41 and 42 in the temporal lobe (related to hearing); areas 1, 2, and 3 in the post central gyrus of the parietal lobe (the somatosensory region); and areas 17 and 18 in the occipital lobe (the primary visual areas).[15] It is noted that

> Brodmann areas were originally defined and numbered based on the organization of neurons he observed in the cortex using the Nissl stain. Brodmann published his maps of cortical areas in humans, monkeys, and other species in 1909, along with many other findings and observations regarding the general cell types and laminar organization of the mammalian cortex. (The same Brodmann area number in different species does not necessarily indicate homologous areas.) Although the Brodmann areas have been discussed, debated, refined, and renamed exhaustively for nearly a century, they remain the most widely known and frequently cited cyto-architectural organization of the human cortex. Many of the areas Brodmann defined

---

[14] http://www.stanford.edu/group/hopes/rltdsci/trinuc/f_f03motrsoma.jpg
[15] http://en.wikipedia.org/wiki/Korbinian_Brodmann

based solely on their neuronal organization have since been correlated closely to diverse cortical functions.[16]

Diagram 7: Brodmann Areas

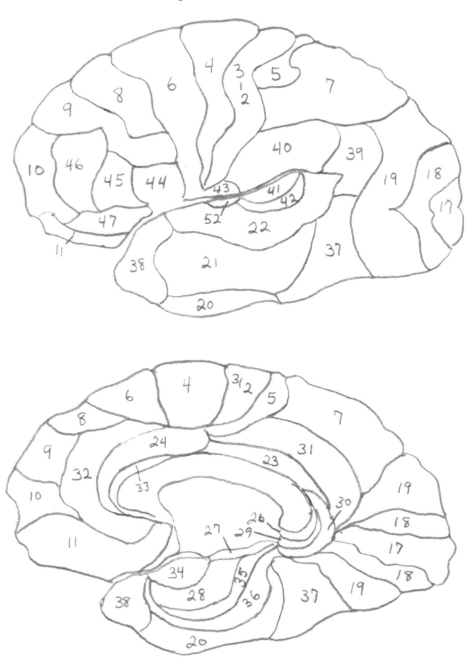

[16] http://en.wikipedia.org/wiki/Brodmann_area

Two basic divisions of cell type in the brain are neurons and glial cells. Neurons provide electro-chemical activity and glial cells provide maintenance and support for the neurons. Neurons provide the 30 watts of power the brain generates to carry out its business. Over the last few years, research has indicated that the glial cells may play more of a role in information processing than previously thought and are far more than just support cells.

The neuron is profoundly complex, and a basic orientation is necessary in order to understand EEG. The neuron can be divided into four basic components: the dendrites, the soma, the axon, and the synapse.

The soma, or cell body, can be thought of as a simple battery that stores electrical energy by maintaining an electrical charge differential between the inside and outside of its cell wall. It connects to several other neurons through a main fiber that runs out of it called an axon. Diagram 8, below, shows an example of a neuron.

Diagram 8: Electrode and Neuron Reception

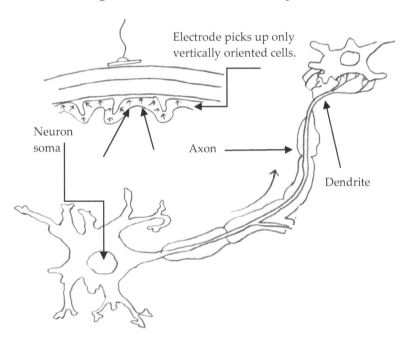

Dendrites are protrusions from the soma that collect electrical signals from several other cell axons. Between the end of each axon and the dendrite of another cell to which it connects is a gap known as the synapse.

The synapse operates like a switch that induces the neuron to fire an electrical impulse. The electrical charge travels down the axon to its own synapse that in turn induces other neurons to fire. This firing is referred to as the action potential. The action potential at the transmitter site is an "all or none" event. There is a rest period during which time the neuron recovers, i.e., rebuilds its charge, called the refractory period. Neurons collect impulses from between 5,000 and 50,000 other neurons. These impulses either encourage or discourage the neuron from firing. When encouraged, they are depolarized. When discouraged, they are hyperpolarized. The entire cycle from depolarization through recovery takes about two milliseconds.

At the end of each axon is a button-shaped terminal that generates chemicals known as neurotransmitters (see Diagram 9: The Synapse). These are contained in sacks known as vesicles, which migrate to the end of the button when a charge arrives. The neurotransmitters release flow across the synaptic gap and settle in receptor sites on the receiving dendrite. Receptor sites may increase or decrease over time in response to the average volume of neurotransmitter activity. If excessive neurotransmitter activity occurs over time, the receptors will reduce their population to adjust for the heavy traffic. Heavy alcohol users, for example, may cause excessive amounts of dopamine to cross gaps, eventually causing receptor populations to reduce. If the alcoholic suddenly stops, too little dopamine will be produced with respect to the existing receptor populations. Motor systems will suffer from reduced efficiency. Consequently, the alcoholic's hand may shake like someone with Parkinson's disease. This same process occurs in the hippocampal switching mechanisms that control immune function in response to cortisol levels generated by stress. Prolonged stress degrades the switching mechanism and immune response may be overactive when the stress lifts.

Diagram 9: The Synapse

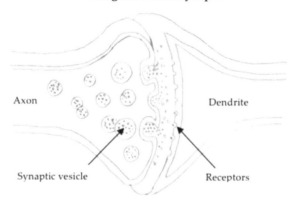

Axon

Dendrite

Synaptic vesicle

Receptors

THE NEUROTRANSMITTER SYSTEMS

Rivers of neurochemical systems flow throughout the brain that help fuel shifts in levels of function in different brain areas by increasing or decreasing synaptic activity that generates EEG frequencies. Neurons tend to specialize in the neurotransmitters they use to communicate with one another, although they may respond to many others. These systems form networks that run throughout the brain. Tribes or clusters of neurons barter in basically one neurotransmitter currency. Sometimes they make exchanges in other currencies. The cerebellar vermis modulates the production and release of neurotransmitters.

The body may have hundreds of neurotransmitters. However, medical science has only isolated around sixty, and medical doctors tend to focus on the ones that have the most general effect. Neuroscience has found that pharmacologically manipulating these neurotransmitters can alter and help regulate basic overall dysfunctions in brain systems. Consequently, it is assumed that neurotransmitters are the basic chemical modulators of brain function. They are referred to as neuromodulators and are further divided into slow- and fast-acting neurotransmitters. (In neuromodulation, several classes of neurotransmitters regulate diverse populations of central nervous system neurons (one neuron uses different neurotransmitters to connect to several neurons). Examples of neuromodulators include dopamine, serotonin, acetylcholine, histamine, and others. The notion of a neuromodulator is a relatively new concept. A neuromodulator can be conceptualized as a neurotransmitter that is not reabsorbed by the pre-synaptic neuron or broken down into a metabolite. Such neuromodulators end up spending a significant amount of time in the cerebrospinal fluid (CSF), influencing (or modulating) the overall activity level of the brain. For this reason, some neurotransmitters are also considered as neuromodulators, such as serotonin and acetylcholine.[17]) Below is a list of these modulators and their related general areas of function (see Table 1: Major Neurotransmitters, below, and DiagramDiagram 10: Norepinephrine System, page 40).

Table 1: Major Neurotransmitters

Neurotransmitters	Type	Source, Major Influence Areas, Associated Disorders
Dopamine	biogenic amine inhibitory	substantia nigra: attentional networks, hedonic centers, schizophrenia, ADHD, addictions
Serotonin	biogenic amine inhibitory	Raphe nuclei: mood centers, sleep cycles depression, addictions
Norepinephrine	biogenic amine excitatory	locus coeruleus: general arousal levels, attentional networks
Acetylcholine	cholinergic	acetylcholine nuclei: memory networks, memory problems
GABA	amino acid inhibitory	global: general arousal levels, anxiety disorders
Histamine	biogenic amine	global

---

[17] http://en.wikipedia.org/wiki/Neuromodulation Retrieved March 12, 2011.

Diagram 10: Norepinephrine System

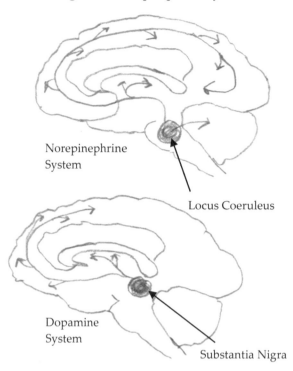

Norepinephrine System

Locus Coeruleus

Dopamine System

Substantia Nigra

THE NEUROTRANSMITTER EEG CONNECTION

An approximate correlation between EEG activity and neurotransmitter activity appears to exist. The two reflect different fundamental levels of activity in the brain. The correlation is not precise. However, there is clearly a functional relationship that is useful to consider, since so much intervention and research is directed toward the neurotransmitter systems. The use of drugs also alters EEG activity; it is important to be aware of this alteration when reading EEG and taking baselines (see Table 2: Drug Effect on EEG, below).

Table 2: Drug Effect on EEG

Drug/Type	Impact/Effect on EEG
Barbiturates	Increase 25-35 Hz beta amplitude
Benzodiazepines	Increase beta
Caffeine	Increases beta and decreases slower waves
Marijuana	Affects EEG for three days by increasing global alpha
SSRIs	Decrease alpha and increase beta

From a neurotherapist's perspective, the attentional network largely drives the entire system once the person is awake and alert. Joel Lubar has voiced similar conclusions. Other than that, it appears to be maintained in systematic equilibrium through iterative cycles by brain stem networks. This is of interest because so much of EEG training involves the attentional networks and much of the work done with ADHD relates to this area as well.

Neurofeedback causes fundamental shifts in neurotransmitter system activity in much the same way that drugs can also be used to alter them. This is not a surprise because any exposure to important stimuli can generate major shifts in EEG as the organism orients to take action. For instance, Ron Ruden (1997) reports that researchers have found a very strong correlation between alpha training and general increases in serotonin.

CORTICAL SYSTEMS: PYRAMIDAL CELLS, CELL COLUMNS, AND LAYERS

The cortex is comprised of groups of cells referred to as cell columns or macrocolumns, which are several millimeters in diameter. These columns are composed of functionally related groups of cells that run vertically through the 6 layers of the cortex (as discussed in Chapter 2). The exact nature of these columns and the area of their physical extension are still under debate.

From an EEG perspective, it is when these columns are in the process of firing together that the wave fronts become recorded as EEG. Nunez (2006) indicates, however, that EEG cannot be used to specifically measure activity at the macrocolumn level of activity. In fact, synchronous activity of about 60,000,000 pyramidal cells or 600,000 macrocolumns is required to generate a readable EEG signal at the scalp. This amount of activity is defined as a single "dipole layer" and is typically 6 cm squared in size. This is roughly half the size of Broca's area.

It should be apparent that traditional EEG measures only broad areas of activity. Therefore, it has limited spatial resolution (as compared to the spatial precision of MRI). The summated dipoles (active current flow around a cell) that generate a dipole layer are from a particular type of cell, a pyramidal cell. It is the pyramidal cell that is most responsible for the generation of the pre- and post-synaptic potentials that end up as EEG (see Diagram 11: Cell Columns, page 42).

Pyramidal cells outnumber all other cell types in the cortex and have a special orientation to the six layers of the cortex. Apical dendrites (dendrites that emerge from the apex of a pyramidal cell) extend vertically through the layers and basal dendrites extend horizontally.

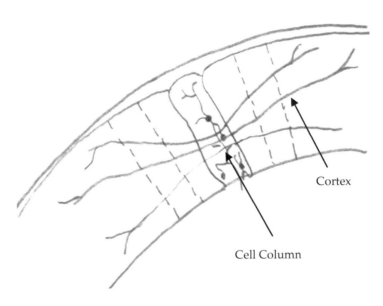

Cortex

Cell Column

The axon of the pyramidal cell extends downward out of the grey matter and becomes part of the white matter (see Diagram 12: Axon and Cell Columns, below). So the input to these cells comes from the upper layers and their output extends downward through their axons. The larger cells exist in the lower layers and occupy layers 2, 3, 5, and 6. Stellate cells[18] help communication between pyramidal cells within the cortex and are called interneurons. They exist mostly in layer 4.

Diagram 12: Axon and Cell Columns

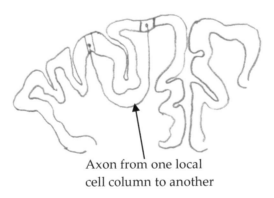

Axon from one local
cell column to another

---

[18] Stellate cells are neurons with several dendrites radiating from the cell bodies, giving them a star-shaped appearance. The three most common stellate cells are the inhibitory interneurons found within the molecular layer of the cerebellum, excitatory spiny stellate interneurons, and inhibitory aspiny stellate interneurons (http://en.wikipedia.org/wiki/Stellate_cell).

Inputs to the cortex come from the thalamus and from other areas of the cortex (association fibers) and enter in layer 6 at the base. Thalamic input fibers generally end in layers 4 and 3. This apparently makes them the main input layers. Association fibers tend to input in layers 6, 5, 3, 2, and 1.

Outputs from cells in layer 6 generally go to the thalamus while those in layer 5 go to subcortical nuclei. Most outputs go to other cortical areas. Layers 2 and 3 generally reinput back to the cortex, so outputs generally go to three areas: cortex, thalamus, and subcortex.

FIBER SYSTEMS

The wiring of the cortex is composed of axons (white matter) that run in bundles along specific pathways. It is important to understand this wiring because it is through these bundles of fibers that areas of the brain are functionally connected for intermodal and cross-modal operations (in QEEG this is referred to as coherence). It is the summation of these operations that generate coordinated behavior and perception. When looking at a brain map, it is easier to understand what areas may be affecting other areas and the consequences of hyper- and hypo-coupling between cell ensembles. Phase and coherence analysis attempts to assess the level of connectivity in these pathways.

There are two basic association subcortical fiber systems (see Diagram 13: Subcortical Fiber Systems, page 44) that are involved with intracortex communication or cortico-cortico (cortex-to-cortex) exchange. The two types include short association fibers, which connect adjacent areas or gyri of the brain, and the long association fibers, which connect more distant regions. There are three basic long association fiber systems. The cingulum is within the cingulate gyrus and connects frontal and parietal lobes with parts of the temporal lobes. The uncinate fasciculus connects the orbital lobe and other parts of the frontal lobe with the anterior temporal lobe. Parts of it also connect with the occipital lobe. The arcurate fasciculus connects parts of the frontal lobe with the temporal lobe as well, especially Broca's area and Wernicke's area, which relate to processing and speaking language in the left hemisphere.

Another fiber system, the commissures, connects the hemispheres and is known as the corpus callosum and the anterior commissure. These fiber systems are concerned with short-term memory functions: the transference of learned tasks between hemispheres. As noted in Chapter 2, severe damage can occur to this area of the brain as the result of child abuse.

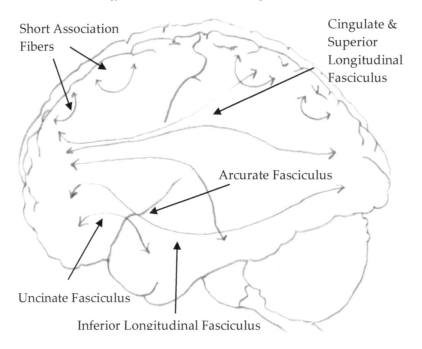

Short Association Fibers

Cingulate & Superior Longitudinal Fasciculus

Arcurate Fasciculus

Uncinate Fasciculus

Inferior Longitudinal Fasciculus

BRODMANN'S AREAS: CONNECTING THE DOTS

As noted above, Brodmann analyzed the brain based on the congregation of cell types in different areas of the brain. These brain areas are frequently used by neurologists to associate function with location. Table 3: Brodmann Areas and Localization of Function on page 46 shows the Brodmann's areas as they relate to function and EEG. The International 10-20 System of electrode placement is shows on Diagram 14: 10-20 System of Electrode Placement, page 45. Today, neuro-imaging is resulting in a new mapping system, but it has not yet been entirely integrated into neurology and neuro-psychology.

PROJECTION TRACTS

The projection tracts are fiber systems that bring information into the cortex from the thalamus as well as output information and are known as the corona radiata. One group of projection tracts connects the frontal cortex to the thalamus. A second group of projection tracts connects to motor neurons through the reticular formation. Another group connects parietal, occipital, and temporal fibers to the spinal cord. Two other groups of projection tracts connect to auditory and optical functions in the temporal and occipital lobes respectively.

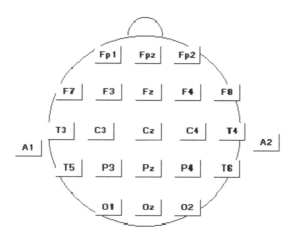

THALAMIC PROJECTION SYSTEM

The thalamus is divided into sections that connect to specific related areas of the brain. These connections are through axons extending to and received from pyramidal cells in the lower layers of the cortex. These axons appear to set up resonances between the thalamus and the cortex. Oscillating neurons in the thalamus send signals in specific frequency ranges to the cortex, which in turn sends feedback to the thalamus. A constant dialogue is established where different sections of the brain engage and disengage as the cortex coordinates its various modules into organized behavior.

Early researchers felt that alpha rhythms were primarily generated by the thalamus alone, but newer theories contend that although alpha does spontaneously emanate from thalamic neuronal oscillator circuits, their shifting patterns are driven through interaction with the cortex. The alpha range represents a functional idling frequency that turns off or "desynchronizes" as different sections of the brain become active. The on-task activity appears to involve gating mechanisms in the beta range. Lower frequency activity in theta appears to be related to resonances with subcortical activities, particularly in the limbic system.

Table 3: Brodmann Areas and Localization of Function

SITE	BRODMANN AREA	FUNCTION
Fpz	10, 11, 32	Emotional inhibition, oversensitive, impulsive Motivation & attention
Fp1	10, 11, 46	Cognitive emotional valence - lateral orbital frontal Irritability, intrusive, depression Social awareness - approach behaviors
Fp2	10, 11, 46	Emotional inhibition - lateral orbital frontal Impulsivity, tactlessness, mania Social awareness - avoidance behaviors
F7	45, 47, 46	Working memory - visual & auditory Divided & selective attention - filtering Broca's area - semantic short-term buffer (word retrieval)
F8	45, 47, 46	Prosody Working memory - spatial & visual, gestalt Facial emotional processing Sustained attention
F3	8, 9, 46	Short-term memory - verbal episodic retrieval Facial recognition, object processing Planning & problem solving - Wisconsin card sort (rigidity)
F4	8, 9, 46	Short-term memory - spatial/object retrieval Vigilance area - selective & sustained attentional area
Fz	8, 6, 9	Personality changes Intention & motivation - poverty of speech, apathy Possible anterior cingulate - internal vs. external attention Basal ganglia output
C3	3, 1, 4	Sensory & motor functions
C4	3, 1, 4	Sensory & motor functions
Cz	6, 4, 3	Sensory & motor functions
T3	42, 22, 21	Language comprehension - verbal understanding Wernicke's area - inner voice Long-term memory - declarative & episodic processing Event sequencing - visualization Amygdala/hippocampal area
T4	42, 22 ,21	Personality - emotional tonality (anger, sadness) Categorization & organization Visualization and auditory cortex
T5	39, 37, 19	Meaning construction - angular gyrus Acalcula Short-term memory
T6	39, 37, 19	Facial recognition - emotional content, amygdalic connection
P3	7, 40, 19	Digit span problems, information organization problems Self-boundaries excessive thinking
P4	7, 40, 19	Visual processing - spatial sketch pad, vigilance Personality - excessive self-concern, victim mentality Agnosia, apraxia, context boundaries, rumination
Pz	7, 5, 19	Attentional shifting- perseverance Self-awareness, orientation association area Agnosia, apraxia
O1, O2	18, 19, 17	Visual processing, procedural memory, dreaming
Oz	18, 17, 19	Visual processing, hallucinations

New Mind Neurofeedback Center

Barry Sterman has pioneered work demonstrating the gating system by which sensory information is directed toward the motor cortex or blocked through thalamic oscillators. As a consequence of these findings, Sterman has experimented with individuals who have seizure disorders. He dramatically reduced the frequency of seizures through SMR training. Joel Lubar (Lubar & Bahler, 1976 later applied these findings with considerable success to individuals with ADHD. Sterman found that seizure activity continued to decline over a period of a decade after patients quit training, while Lubar found, in likewise fashion, that individuals with ADHD continued to show improvement after training as well.

NEOCORTICAL DYNAMICS: OSCILLATORS, WAVEFRONTS, AND NETWORKS

OSCILLATORS

Oscillators are groups of neurons that work together to generate rhythmic pulses of electrical activity. According to Buzsaki (2006), they form momentary cohorts of activity, called cell assemblies, networking together for 30-100ms or more. They are associated physiologically with glucose and oxygen consumption and neurometabolic coupling, which is controlled by local cells called astrocytes (Freeman, Ahlfors, & Menon, 2009). Oscillatory circuits are in both the cortex and the thalamus.

Theories of how EEG arises and propagates itself are still evolving. The EEG at the surface of the cortex (see Diagram 15: EEG Wavefronts, page 48) reflects the summated activity of ensembles of cells in the form of extracellular current flow. This summated activity is due apparently to synchronously activated postsynaptic potentials from vertically oriented pyramidal cells. Nunez (1995) proposes that this summated activity forms standing wavefronts that hover over the surface of the cortex and scalp. According to his calculations, these wavefronts are so large that there is no neutral site to place a reference electrode that would allow for an approximately infinite resistance between the wave sources required for a true reference site. Thus, the ear lobes have been chosen as common reference points for databases as a good compromise (rather than the nose, another good compromise).

The contribution to the EEG recorded at a specific site has been theoretically determined by Nunez (1995) and involves the following definition:

$$f(n), b\ (BQ)$$

where
f = frequencies,
n = spatial patterns (corresponding frequencies and overtones);

b = multiple frequencies in the same medium interacting;
B = global control parameters (neurotransmitter activity);
and Q = local control parameters (physical electrical activities causing state transitions).

A simpler heuristic comes from the neurology community and suggests that approximately 40% or more of the total global EEG, or volume-conducted EEG, is being recorded at any given electrode location.

Diagram 15: EEG Wavefronts

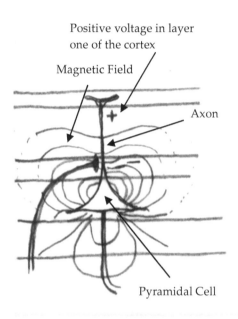

Clearly the area of approximately three square centimeters (approximately the size of a quarter) of activity monitored by an electrode draws its characteristics from a complex mixture of local and distant activity. Consequently, local activity is merely a peculiar reflection of the sum of activity occurring in the brain at that moment. To assume that the activity noted is primarily a reflection of the local activity would be erroneous. To assume that distant activity is or is not affected by local recruitment of EEG is an unsound conclusion. To consider local recruitment to be affecting primarily the local area is equally unsound. Nunez (1995) notes that the complexity of the EEG is such that we do not at present have the mathematical models to untangle it.

In terms of EEG training, this has important implications. Texts on neurology clearly state that the impact of any one area of the brain on others is so complex as to be difficult to untangle in any given situation. These texts rely primarily on the physical behavior of the organism to determine what sections of the brain are most impacted by focal lesions. They find it difficult to predict the specific consequences of damage to one area of the brain. This is also in part due to the great variance in the anatomy of individual function location. This causes difficulties in averaging site findings in functional MRI research as well (however, EEG can invalidate MRI, and PET and functional MRI (fMRI) provides better resolution than EEG and magnetoencephalography [MEG]).

The most recent research involves mathematical simulations based on Hagmann's (2008) mapping of the hubs, nodes, and pathways of the cortex. These simulations are correlated with MRI and anatomical observations of real head injury cases. They indicate that damage to hubs and nodes has more extensive impact than damage to any other areas and the effects on those areas that are secondarily impacted are complex in pattern and difficult to predict (Alstott, Breakspear, Hagmann, Cammoun, & Sporns, 2009). Since hubs and nodes only occupy a relatively small area of the cortex, lesions may frequently have only local consequences but on occasion very extensive bilateral consequences. In light of this, it may be dangerous to assume that training EEG in one specific site will affect all individuals with similar problems in the exact same manner.

The problem becomes even greater when DSM diagnoses are relied on to guide intervention, since they are based on constellations of general behavior patterns rather than specific behaviors used as cues by neurologists. Furthermore, multiple subtypes in terms of EEG with respect to many of the DSM diagnostic categories have been found. For instance, Chabot (1998) believes he has isolated eleven subtypes of ADHD and other researchers have reported five possible subtypes of schizophrenia.

Quantitative EEG brain mapping can indicate abnormal brain function in a specific location using a dynamic electrophysiological perspective. QEEG cannot, however, predict behavioral deviance with accuracy as yet and may never be capable of this, although general categories of EEG constellation have been found highly correlated with specific DSM categories of disorder. New Mind Technologies is presently involved with a collaborative project with the University of North Carolina to collect data comparing dimensions of social behavior with dimensions of QEEG analysis. We expect some predictive relationships to emerge. It should be kept in mind that training based solely on QEEG does not guarantee results. Training at a specific site may not permanently alter activity in that site. On the other hand, it may alter activity, but predicting its effects on other more distant sites is not possible. Therefore, a general catalogue of training patterns for different symptoms may prove more effective in guiding training—although QEEG interpretation may be most effective in determining the general problem from an EEG perspective.

Often, professionals will ask, how does EEG compare to other measures?

9) EEG can invalidate MRI.

10) PET and fMRI provide better spatial resolution than EEG and MEG (magnetoencephalography), but poorer temporal resolution. MRI shows responses in terms of seconds while EEG shows responses in terms of milliseconds.

GLOBAL, REGIONAL, & LOCAL ACTIVITY

Wavefronts can develop as a result of activity involving small local areas as well as multiple areas covering the entire brain. These wavefronts resonate back and forth between various regions of the brain depending on their phase relationships and have come to be referred to as resonant loops. Researchers have divided this activity into three categories: local, regional, and global resonant loops.

The first type of resonant loop is called a local resonant loop and takes place between local cell columns that are known as macro columns (see cortical systems above). There is a great deal of resistance between adjacent cell columns. The brain carefully regulates interaction between local cell columns to avoid too much excitation and seizure activity. In fact, the brain has powerful inhibitory mechanisms in place and much of the electrical activity is dedicated to inhibition. It appears that the brain is delicately balanced between seizure and coma.

The resonances between local cell columns usually occur at frequencies above 30 Hz and are often called gamma. They are beyond the range of present-day QEEG databases. Much of the activity in this frequency range has been associated with excessive mental chatter and disorders such as schizophrenia. It is also the range of a great deal of scalp EMG. It is often difficult to distinguish between gamma and scalp tension. In fact, many researchers believe it is difficult, if not impossible, to increase the amplitude of this frequency range significantly through training.

Resonances around 38-42 Hz are known as Sheer rhythms (Friedemann et al., 1994; Sheer, 1976) and appear to be related to learning. Rhythms of 40 Hz are also thought to be related to activation processes associated with DC current activity in the brain that involves consciousness.

Resonances that develop between cortical cell columns that are several centimeters apart are called regional resonances. The exchange of communication between cortico-cortico sites would also dominate this range as well as cortico-thalamic sites. These resonances result in alpha and low beta activity. It appears that these involve the idling and engagement of cell columns as they process information incoming as a result of attentional activities and conscious articulation.

Global resonances develop as a result of activity between distant sites of the cortex and fall into the theta and delta range. Many of the sites involved in this frequency range are believed to include subcortical functions. Hippocampal-septal activity in the limbic system is known to generate a significant amount of theta activity. Theta activity is associated with co-ordination of cortical networks, memory, and emotional processing as well (Buzsaki, 2006). Presently, it appears that gamma activity, by exciting cortical cell assemblies, is coordinated through timing mechanisms that are associated with theta and may provide a basis for understanding the "binding" mechanisms in the brain.

Robert Thatcher (personal communication) argues that these global resonances are related to meta-functions such as personality functions that are integrative in nature. In addition, we know that theta involves daydreaming and rumination activities. These may be more primitive forms of processing related to subcortical functions. Delta's primary function appears to be related to sleep, yet it is very much a part of waking cortical activity. Although it is in the background, research in QEEG suggests that lack of delta may indicate a lack of continuity in white matter fibers, which could be thought of as low connectivity between networks.

The pattern below (Diagram 16, below) is adopted from Nunez's (1995) book on neocortical dynamics and shows the theoretical pattern of expanding EEG waves generated from local sources over fractions of a second.

Diagram 16: Expanding EEG Waves

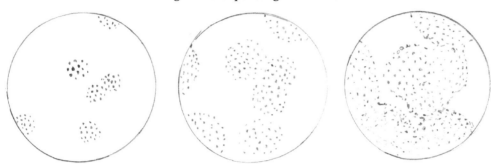

These patterns tend to establish relatively stable patterns that last longer and are called standing waves. The patterns in Diagram 17, below are characteristic of those found during an alpha baseline. They indicate stereotypical patterns of high and low amplitude locations seen in a brain map and may reflect the patterns of neural network activation.

Diagram 17: Stereotypical Patterns of High and Low Amplitude Locations

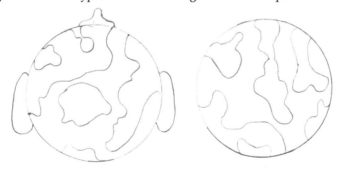

HYPER-COUPLING, HYPO-COUPLING, AND COHERENCE

The resonant loops we have discussed appear to favor different frequencies based on the number of resident synapses and the amount of delay characteristically involved with those neurons. Hypo-coupling in the brain involves smaller loops and higher frequencies.[19] It, therefore,

---

[19] Hypo-coupling involves smaller loops and higher frequencies; higher frequencies are indicative of anxiety and seizure (norepinephrine, dopamine); hyper-coupling is said to occur when brain activation decreases, slow waves increase, serotonin levels drop, and depression and impulsivity increase.

characterizes a high level of cerebral activation and arousal that is often reflected in conscious or awake information processing states. As the brain becomes engaged in hyper-coupled activity, activation decreases and slow wave activity increases while the brain moves toward an increased resting state and sleep.

Too much hypo-coupling moves us toward excess activity, anxiety, and seizure. Too much hyper-coupling moves us toward reduced activity, depression, impulsivity, and coma. Excessive hypo-coupling shows up in positive schizophrenia and anxiety with excessive activity in the 23-38 Hz range. Excessive hyper-coupling is found in negative schizophrenia and ADHD with excessive activity in the 1 Hz to 8 Hz range. Increasing the average level of activity in the 9 Hz to 15 Hz range to reduce activity in the upper and lower frequency ranges is often an important goal of training.

Coherence describes the relationship between two localities in the brain. As cell ensembles fire and generate wavefronts, their frequencies often match up as they resonate together. The more they resonate together, the more their timing becomes synchronized. The peaks and valleys of their waveforms begin to match each other and they become phase locked. When the two waves become perfectly overlapped we say they are synchronous (see diagramDiagram 18: Wavelength and Phase, below). This is a special case of coherence, and is referred to as state phase coherence in electronics theory. The peaks and valleys of the waves match up in lock step.

When the peaks and valleys of the waves match up in lock step, their phase angle becomes zero. The degree to which they phase lock is often spoken of in terms of an average phase angle. When locations are 180 degrees out of phase, their peaks are occurring at opposite times. In neurometrics, coherence refers to the degree in which two locations have a consistent phase angle. When their phase angle is consistent, they are considered to be in a high level of communication. When coherence is too high, there is a lack of differentiation between functional areas. When coherence is low, there is a lack of communication between functional areas.

Diagram 18: Wavelength and Phase

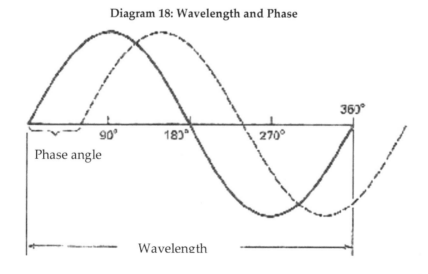

Technically, the whole issue is more complex, and there is considerable disagreement in the definition of EEG coherence. EEG coherence is formally defined as the co-variation of phase over time with respect to a mean value based on a database. According to Duane Shuttlesworth (personal communication), the late E. Roy John chose the definition of covariance of power between various sites in the left and right hemispheres. To confuse issues more, Sterman has introduced a similar measure he calls comodulation, which is the covariance of frequency over time with respect to a mean value based on a database.

At this point, Nunez (2006) indicates that coherence measures are highly contaminated by volume conduction over interelectrode distances of up to 10 cm. This would invalidate a large portion of the connections displayed on the average QEEG. Roberto Pascual Marqui (2007), who developed Low Resolution Tomography (LORETA) imaging at the Key Institute, echoes these concerns in his latest research and argues that coherence is a two-dimensional measurement. David Kaiser, who co-developed the Sterman Kaiser Database, goes further and says that it is one dimensional (personal communication). He also indicates that two-dimensional coherence is confounded by possible contributions from a third-dimensional source involving thalamic mediation (personal communication). David Kaiser and Paul Nunez argue that coherence should be based on Laplacian transforms to be accurate. Thatcher argues that this practice only distorts phase measures upon which coherence is based. Taking these arguments into account, it may be best to consider coherence as a vague but general measure of connectivity.

Phase is defined as the degree to which the peak and trough cycles of two sites agree, what is often referred to as phase angle in electronics. Coherence is derived from phase since it measures how consistent this relationship is over time. Symmetry, on the other hand, is the covariance of amplitude at two different sites. Training coherence and phase differences between two locations is becoming popular, especially with traumatic brain injury (TBI) and learning disabilities (LD), even though there is little research on the topic. Jonathan Walker, a neurologist from Texas, is one of the leading proponents and most experienced clinicians in this area. Several manufacturers have begun to offer equipment with two or more channels that have this capability. It should be noted that we have pre and post brain maps showing major changes from coherence due to training in the amplitude (magnitude) domain. One domain affects the other domain (i.e., power or magnitude has an effect on coherence and coherence has an effect on power). The research question that needs to be answered regards the advantages that might be gained by training coherence. Although coherence and power (or magnitude) are mathematically different and independent dimensions, functionally they are not different. The brain is a dynamic system that derives power and magnitude as a consequence of phase activity (Srinivasan & Nunez, 2006).

BrainMaster Technlogies has developed a new approach to training using a DLL (dynamic linked library) to link live EEG training to the Neuroguide database. This new technology is referred to as "Z score training." This method allows coherence to be trained within specific parameters based on the normative database. This assures that coherence will be trained within very carefully defined limits, so that it cannot easily be trained too high or too low. As coherence training has become more popular, many clinicians have noted serious unintended side effects. The Z-score training method appears to minimize this problem.

The Othmers have proposed that their new protocol techniques result in a form of "anti-coherence training" that encourages plasticity in networks that are too high in coherence. Siegfried has also indicated that they may move from the bipolar montages. They presently use a two-channel version of this approach that might be more precise and controlled. Currently, however, the Othmers are doing sub-delta training.

COMODULATION

Barry Sterman and David Kaiser have developed the connectivity measure known as comodulation. It is mathematically derived from the covariance of power of two electrode locations. This measure looks at the correlation of magnitude between locations. Although it is not presently represented in other database systems, it appears to be a very valuable correlate of disorder and capable of predicting specific functional problems. There is not very much research employing this measure at present, but it may prove more robust than coherence in the future.

CONNECTIVITY

Connectivity is a hot topic in neurofeedback and QEEG at present. Many arguments surround issues regarding what are the best measures of connectivity and how to obtain and represent them. Freeman (2009) defines connectivity along two dimensions: effective and functional. Functional connectivity indicates the actual existing integration of hubs, nodes, and networks at baseline or rest. Effective connectivity concerns how well modules and networks communicate "under load" or during a task. This difference is reflected in a baseline EEG vs. EEG during training. A QEEG typically shows functional connectivity unless it is done during a task, such as reading. A healthy EEG distribution during a resting QEEG indicates good functional connectivity with respect to the default mode of operation. This important emerging research in the neuroimaging community profoundly validates the use of both QEEG as an assessment measure and neurofeedback as a remedial intervention.

The most recent efforts in the development of many EEG database systems is to develop a three-dimensional measure of connectivity, such as Hudspeth's Neurorep System (see REFER TO SECTION IN CHAP. 2) and the Key Institute's LORETA (See refer to section in chap 2). There may be mathematical, spatial, and temporal limits to this agenda. Thatcher is focusing more on measuring network configurations based on phase locking, which appears to be a more realistic solution. The New Mind database system, on the other hand, focuses instead on EEG as a measure of activation and uses multivariate analysis to determine this dimension. This is more in line with the present approach of the neuroimaging community and is grounded in 100 years of postmortem studies and clinical observations in neurology.

In reviewing the literature on connectivity, key concepts emerge from Buzsaki's (2006) analysis regarding connectivity.

Connectivity is Reciprocal

- Network hierarchy is determined by computational solution - i.e., no real top and bottom solution.

- Function is highly distributive.
- Synaptic weighting emerges from auto-associative attractor networks.
- All circuits can sustain autonomous self-organizing activity.
- Connectivity is a combination of modular and small world activity.
- Not all routes are equal between neurons.
- Gamma synchrony is the key to network activation over long distances.
- Order is a function of environmental attachment.

All of these issues must be ultimately taken into account when analyzing connectivity. Clearly this is a long-term project for the QEEG community and will not be resolved in the near future. This should guide us to be cautious when we evaluate any claims made with regard to the representation of connectivity.

TRADITIONAL BANDWIDTHS

Traditionally the EEG spectrum is divided into bandwidths with the names alpha, beta, theta, and delta. (Alpha is further broken down into lo-alpha and hi-alpha, and beta is further broken down into lo-beta, beta, and hi-beta). In the past, these have been used as if they were the only possible ones to consider, although others such as gamma were discussed. The waves in these bandwidths have a specific shape or morphology that helped to identify them. Electroencephalographers traditionally count the number of wave peaks in a second and look at the wave shape to identify the wave type they are viewing. So there are two components to the analysis: frequency and morphology. Most people in neurofeedback tend to rely mostly on frequency. This can be misleading at times, especially with respect to alpha because alpha can be as slow as 3 Hz or as fast as 15 Hz and is primarily identified by morphology. Below are some samples of typical wave types. To learn them all requires considerable study. Courses in EEG technology are offered at local colleges and can be helpful to gain a better understanding of EEG.

The first wave type presented is rhythmic delta (Diagram 19: Rhythmic Delta, below) and is usually considered to be from 1.5 to 3.5 or 1 to 4 cycles per second. It is a normal type of delta you would expect to find in your EEG and is predominantly present in deep sleep. The second type of delta is non-rhythmic and is abnormal (see Diagram 20: Non-rhythmic Delta, page 56). It is often present when individuals move their eyes around or shift around in their seats. It may also be present in areas with white matter lesions. According to Robert Thatcher (personal communication), and based on his research with EEG and MRI, high levels of localized delta on a brain map may indicate white matter damage as well.

Diagram 19: Rhythmic Delta

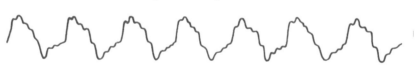

Diagram 20: Non-rhythmic Delta

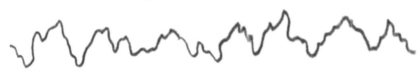

The next sample is rhythmic theta and irregular theta (Diagram 21 and 22, below). Rhythmic theta is a normal variant that is present in the waking EEG and is found in a bandwidth between 3.5 and 7.5 or 4 and 7 cycles a second. You will often see it increase as individuals get drowsy or start daydreaming while training. Five cycles per second theta has been found to be associated with memory functions. According to Thatcher (personal communication), high amplitude focal theta may be associated with damage to the cortex. Theta spikes are common when individuals blink. This can be a problem for eyes-open training, especially in front of the motor strip.

Diagram 21: Rhythmic Theta

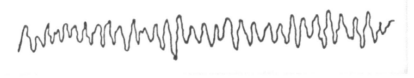

Diagram 22: Non-rthymic Theta

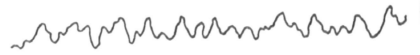

Diagram 23: Normal Alpha Wave, below, shows the smooth-flowing EEG pattern of the alpha wave. It resides generally in a frequency band between 7.5 and 12.5 cycles per second (or 8-12 Hz). Alpha may go as low as 3 cycles per second according to Frank Duffy (1989). Recent research by Hughes and Crunelli (2005) supports this position as well. Many medically trained professionals consider the alpha spectrum to go as high as 14 cycles per second. When 14 Hz hi alpha occurs over the motor strip, it becomes SMR. This sample waxes and wanes in what looks slightly like spindles. This is common in alpha. Alpha represents the brain in a resting or neutral state, yet it is prepared for action. It is often referred to as the idling frequency.

Diagram 23: Normal Alpha Wave

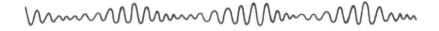

The low-amplitude rapidly fluctuating sample in Diagram 24, page 57, shows the beta wave. It is sometimes called desynchronized EEG. It is frequently considered any frequency above alpha and indicates cortical processing. We see beta occur when people problem solve or think carefully about a topic. When individuals worry constantly, it appears in higher amplitudes. It takes the brain a great deal of energy to produce these higher frequencies, so they tend to always be lower in amplitude than the lower frequencies. Their amplitude is further attenuated more than lower frequencies as they pass through the skull and scalp. According to Marvin Sams (personal communication), real beta occurs in spindles. If it does not, then it is artifact. Continuous sinusoidal beta that is focal may be a lack of inhibitory control over an area.

Diagram 24: Typical Spindling Beta Wave

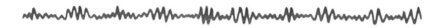

Finally, there is a sample of abnormal waveforms known as sharp waves and spikes (see Diagram 25, below). These waves may often be associated with seizure activity. They are both usually very high in amplitude and fairly random in their occurrence. The spike is very narrow, whereas sharp waves tend to be a little wider.

Diagram 25: Sharp Waves and Spikes

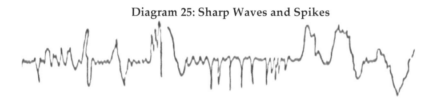

This section has been a brief review of what is frequently referred to as morphology of waveforms. Amplitudes and frequency are considered in the spectral analysis often focused on in neurofeedback, but morphology is often overlooked. Important clues can come from the EEG wave shapes themselves regarding organic problems. Jay Gunkleman provides regular and valuable workshops on this topic.

NONLINEAR DYNAMICS AND EEG

It is clear that the brain maintains a careful balance between seizure and coma. Most of its activity is inhibitory in nature. A contained maelstrom delicately balanced would be a good description. Seizures often appear like thunderstorms or spreading wildfires in the brain. The brain appears to maintain its balance between hypo- and hyper-coupling by constantly returning to a balanced state centered around 10 Hz while performing waking activity (also known as Berger rhythm). This center is so robust that individuals never deviate from a mean resting alpha of 10 Hz by more than .5 Hz on average. The standard deviation from the mean of 10 Hz is, therefore, .5 Hz. This is a very tight range. Sterman's research with pilots reveals that too much average time outside this range exhausts individuals. Their task performance level degrades quickly. For instance, individuals suffering from depression often have an average alpha frequency of around

7 Hz or 8 Hz. These individuals can barely perform. It is clear that their neurotransmitter systems are severely depleted, possibly from too long a period in hypo-coupled states of anxiety.

Theories of nonlinear dynamics state that complex systems move through iterations or cycles, which are so complex that their patterns are very difficult to determine. They appear to be almost random, yet a high level of order is maintained over long periods of time. These systems usually have at least one center of focus or balance, or attractor state, through which they maintain continuity and reference. Whirlpools in a stream are a good example. Although there are complex current flows, the whirlpool remains fairly stable in configuration and location. By using this model for EEG activity, it is easy to draw a correlation between 10 Hz alpha and the attractor state postulated in nonlinear dynamics theory. It has been proposed that this attractor state reflects the health of the entire system and that dysregulation leads to more average time away from this standing attractor state in the brain. This theory is somewhat supported by Sterman's research and the work of David McCormick (1999), Hughes and Crunelli (2005), Silberstein (Nunez, 1995), and other clinical observations.

Ron Ruden (1997) also proposes that the brain, as a consequence of stress and trauma, actually grows networks that lead to progressively more dysregulation and greater deviance from the existing attractor state. This dysregulation generates greater noise in the system and consequently more dysfunctional behavior. This generates a shift in the attractor state that Ruden calls neohomeostasis. Neohomeostasis, therefore, reflects an actual physical growth of dendrites, which generates an organic abnormality in the brain with respect to its intended pattern of development. New neural networks contributing to such a new configuration may involve closed loops that protect the neohomeostasis and may be reflected in obsessional rumination patterns and delusional thinking. Recent articles by David McCormick (1999) also suggest that dysrhythmias causing shifts in the normal functioning of thalamocortical loops lead to disorder. In addition, the work of Joseph LeDoux (1996) indicates that old networks never die, but that new inhibitory networks need to be grown to alter and manage these "networks of trauma."

NEUROTRANSMITTER SYSTEMS AND EEG CORRELATES

Given the frequency with which drugs are employed to deal with psychological problems, it is often considerably beneficial to know their effects on the brain and EEG. The first step in understanding this is to be aware of the relationship between neurotransmitters and EEG. The primary neuromodulators are usually the main focus of drug interventions. In particular, dopamine, serotonin, and GABA are frequently targeted systems (although GABA is a fast-acting neurotransmitter). Much of the work correlating EEG and neurotransmitters is still highly theoretical, but the research so far points towards a pattern that has been proposed as a model. Nunez's book (1995) provides a model favored by Lubar in which serotonin levels drop as the brain moves toward hyper-coupling and slows down. Acetylcholine, norepinephrine, and dopamine activities are correlated with hypo-coupling and increased activity. Consequently, alpha occupies the optimal coupling range while movement toward theta reflects hyper-coupling and movement toward beta reflects hypo-coupling. Diagram 18: Wavelength and Phase, page 52, demonstrates this concept.

Using this model of the brain being driven by attentional networks, we propose that the brain's orientation towards a stimulus is driven by dopamine increases in the nucleus accumbens, which generates excitement in the norepinephrine system (shift to high alpha). This in turn reduces GABA levels and increases activation in sectors of the brain used to process that stimulus object (beta processing). At the same time, acetylcholine is increasing to drive the memory systems so comparator functions can take place (5-6 Hz theta activity increases). Serotonin levels begin to rise to accommodate the increases in the entire system. As behavior brings closure to the attentional cycle, serotonin keeps the brakes on the whole system through its large inhibitory network. Once closure is achieved, serotonin levels slowly drop back as the system returns to biological homeostasis. If orientation and activity happen too frequently and the system becomes overdriven (as in long periods of stressful over-arousal), then norepinephrine depletion occurs and serotonin levels drop to shut the system down (alpha depression). This shutdown will remain protectively in place until environmental cues (internal or external in humans) indicate that chronic aggravation of the system will not reoccur.

Sometimes the gas pedal gets stuck, resulting in chronic high dopamine levels associated with mania and schizophrenia. Sometimes the brake pedal gets stuck, resulting in low serotonin levels associated with depression and negative schizophrenia. Anxiety emerges as a consequence of a chronically over-activated GABA system that becomes entrenched early in the chronic over-arousal cycle and remains constant in specific sectors of the cortex even as depression "sets in." In children, it is now known that chronic levels of stress result in cortisol depletion.

HEMISPHERIC DOMINANCE AND EEG

Past research shows that there are normative patterns of bilateral amplitude (Thompson & Thompson, 2003; Davidson, 1995). An amplitude or frequency asymmetry can have significance. Alpha tends to be highest in the right hemisphere while beta tends to dominate in the left. It is unclear what role theta plays in this picture, but having a roughly equivalent theta in both hemispheres appears to be the favored position at present. Lubar (1991) has observed that individuals with high theta do show differences in behavior and disorderly features. Too much theta on the left tends to result in lack of organization, while too much theta on the right results in impulsivity. According to the research of Richard Davidson (2000), the left hemisphere appears to be related to approach behaviors and the right hemisphere to avoidant behaviors. Too little alpha in the right hemisphere correlates with negative behaviors associated with patterns of social withdrawal. Individuals with depression appear to have this pattern. Too much beta on the right is highly correlated with mania as well.

There is also a pattern of EEG from front to back. Fast waves dominate frontally while slow waves dominate occipitally. Most of the brain maps have reflected an EEG spectral pattern similar to that found at Cz except the spectrum shifts toward the fast waves going frontally and toward the slow waves going occipitally. Consequently, theta is still highest at Pz. Individuals with ADHD tend to have too much theta in the front. Depression tends to appear as too much alpha frontally.

When individuals have more than one disorder, the brain may have asymmetries left to right and front to back, resulting in the appearance of four quadrants of asymmetry, as shown in the NxLink QEEG map segments displayed in Diagram 26: Asymmetrics, below.

Each globe represents the head as seen if you are looking down from above. The top of each globe is the front of the head and the bottom is the back, so in cognitive disabilities (learning disability–LD), excessive high amplitude delta is higher in the back than in the front. With ADHD, excess theta is higher in the front and tapers into normal range moving toward the back. Depression appears as high amplitude alpha in the center or the front. Anxiety can appear as excess beta in the front or the back. (see diagram 26, below).

Diagram 26: Asymmetrics

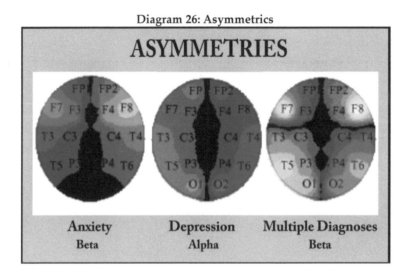

ADDITION POINTS TO NOTE:

- Two-instrument artifact is a condition where two different devices, such as EDR and EEG, are used in the same location. When the electrodes are too close, the result is electrical contamination that distorts the signals being detected by both devices.
- Optical isolation is used in some equipment to enhance safety and reduce artifact. Typically the signal is processed through a pre-amplifier, converted into light, and sent through a fiber optic cable that uses a short optical path to transfer the signal to the main amplifier while keeping it electrically isolated. Since the electrical signal is converted to a light beam, transferred, then converted back to an electrical signal, there is no need for electrical connection between the source and destination circuits.
- EEG alpha asymmetry refers to the observation that alpha is typically higher in magnitude in the right hemisphere than in the left. This is usually an enduring condition that indicates an individual with a stable and positive affect, but nevertheless can reverse itself when such an individual experiences a temporary negative mood. Individuals who chronically experience negative moods usually demonstrate alpha higher in the left hemisphere than in the right.
- REM sleep characterized by sudden eye movement and EMG.

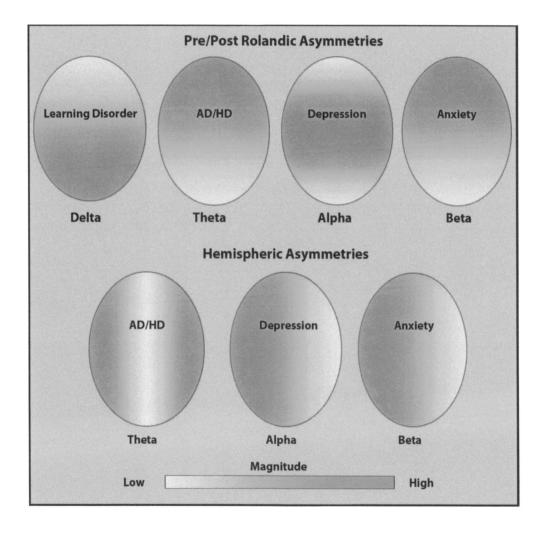

Review Questions

11) What is the Berger rhythm?

12) Brodmann is best known for the development of what system?

13) What system is used for electrode placement?

14) What is an action potential?

15) Can EEG invalidate MRI?

16) Do PET and functional MRI provide better space and resolution than EEG and MEG?

17) What produces EEG alpha asymmetry?

18) What constitutes REM sleep?

19) What is neurometrics?

Chapter Two provided an overview of the brain. Chapter Three provided a brief overview of brainwaves. This chapter takes that information a step further to expand the understanding of how to use QEEG to help validate a patient's diagnosis or self-reported symptoms.

THE SPECTRUM MODEL OF DISORDERS

The dominant emerging model of disorders from an EEG perspective was probably first elucidated by Siegfried Othmer (Evans & Abarbanel, 1999). The model used in our clinics, and through the New Mind Center's QEEG website *New Mind Maps*,[20] is very similar, although derived separately from our own research. We discovered the Othmers' theory after we had developed our own formulation and were surprised to find similarities. We have found several other clinicians who have also arrived at similar conclusions through their own work; however, at this point in the field's evolution it is our belief that before engaging in the use of NFB with patients, the clinician should first conduct some form of QEEG. While QEEG cannot diagnose a particular condition or mental/physical health concern, QEEG can in fact verify a particular diagnosis or verify the reported symptoms of a patient (differential diagnosis).

For example, it has been recognized for some time that excessive dopamine levels and high levels of beta, especially in the 23-38 Hz region, characterize positive schizophrenia. Conversely low dopamine levels and excessive theta in the 4 to 8 Hz range characterize negative schizophrenia. Symptomology of negative schizophrenia and depression are very similar, as are that of positive schizophrenia and anxiety. When reviewing the co-morbidity patterns of disorders, it is apparent that they cluster together in patterns, which further supports the notion that they may not be entirely separate. What many of us see are constellations of symptoms that uniquely reflect the genetic weaknesses in individual systems. These symptoms emerge when the brain is operating too fast or too slow (see Diagram 29: Brain Too Fast and Brain Too Slow on page 70.

Consequently, disorders are placed tentatively along a spectrum in a pattern that appears to be emerging from clinical experience. Anxiety disorders, mania, and OCD show up as excessive frontal fast-wave activity while depression, ADHD, and Tourette's syndrome are associated with excessive frontal slow-wave activity. The specific features of these disorders will be discussed in a later section but Diagram 30 shows a general model (page 71).

 Brain Too Fast: The red shaded area on the left shows the front of the brain as being overactive and producing too much *beta*.

---

[20] https://www.newmindmaps.com/

Brain Too Slow: The red shaded area on the right shows the front of the brain as being underactive (especially the left side) and producing too much *alpha*. We have concluded from our clinical experience that much of the depression we see is end-stage anxiety. Most depressed individuals have experienced elevated levels of anxiety for years and have depleted their neurotransmitter systems (see Chapter Three), to the point where the brain is shutting down to protect itself, hence the high-amplitude, low-frequency alpha. This is congruent with the research on learned helplessness and agrees with the research of Joseph LeDoux (1996).

Many neurotherapists tend to treat symptomology or EEG features rather than DSM categories because the categories don't always correlate with EEG features. As previously mentioned, we often find that there are several EEG subtypes for each category of behavioral disorder. Behavioral typologies and EEG do not always agree. For instance, an individual may score very high on the Beck Depression Inventory and have either excessively high-amplitude, low-frequency alpha 8-9 Hz or excessively high-amplitude, high-frequency alpha 11-14 Hz (anxiety, exhaustion, moving toward entrenched depression). The most effective protocol may be different for different individuals, even though each individual may have depression. Our model of the spectrum of disorders break down as shown below.

TRAUMA AND ITS IMPACT ON THE BRAIN

Reviewing all the available literature on QEEG is beyond the scope of this book. However, there are some basic principles and scientific findings that we would like to review to make the use and comprehension of QEEG more practical from a clinical perspective.

The brain is often negatively impacted when a person is traumatized. Trauma can result from a variety of experiences, which include, but are not limited to the following:

- actual physical injury to the head or traumatic brain injury (TBI)
- neglect, physical abuse, sexual abuse
- exposure to traumatic events such as the death of a sibling or parent, the killing of a family pet or farm animal, natural disasters, life-threatening experiences, and others

Teicher (2007) notes that abuse during childhood, particularly childhood sexual abuse, is a risk factor for development of impulse control disorders, and can lead to a cycle of violence and perpetration. Early stress can exert enduring effects on brain development that may underlie many of the consequences of sexual abuse. Research also shows the negative effects of childhood sexual abuse on development of the hippocampus, corpus callosum, prefrontal cortex, and visual cortex.

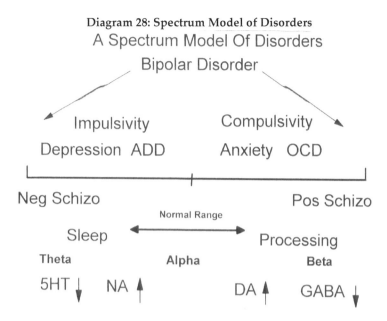

Diagram 28: Spectrum Model of Disorders

A Spectrum Model Of Disorders

Bipolar Disorder

Impulsivity   Compulsivity

Depression ADD   Anxiety OCD

Neg Schizo   Pos Schizo

Normal Range

Sleep   Processing

Theta   Alpha   Beta

5HT ↓   NA ↑   DA ↑   GABA ↓

The Training & Research Institute, Inc. (2004) in Albuquerque, New Mexico, notes that childhood physical, emotional, and sexual abuse and neglect can cause antisocial behavior by over-excitation of the limbic system, the primitive midbrain region that regulates memory and emotion, and the prefrontal cortex, which is associated with judgment, consequential thinking, and moral reasoning. They note the following seven points:

20) The left hemisphere is responsible for regulation and oversight of logical responses to a situation and control and mediation of emotional responses generated by the right hemisphere.

> The impact of childhood abuse or neglect results in diminished control of emotional response, resulting in poor or inappropriate reactions to emotional situations, angry outbursts, self-destructive or suicidal impulses, paranoia, psychosis, and a tendency to pursue intense ultimately unstable relationships.

21) The prefrontal cortex is the internal editor of emotional states, consequential thinking, moral reasoning, and reactions to emotional crisis.

> The impact of childhood abuse or neglect results in increased potential for depression and delinquent and criminal behavior.

22) The corpus collosum creates communication between the right and left hemispheres.

> The impact of childhood abuse or neglect results in a significantly smaller corpus collosum, causing nonintegrated, inappropriate responses to everyday situations. (The larger the corpus collosum, the more one is in contact with their emotions.)

23) The temporal lobes regulate emotions and verbal memory.

> The impact of childhood abuse or neglect results in poor modulation of emotions, and an increased chance for temporal lobe epilepsy.

24) The hippocampus (part of the limbic system) is responsible for the formulation and retrieval of verbal and emotional memories.

> The impact of childhood abuse or neglect results in lower performance on verbal memory tests, possible continued mental problems, and concerns during the adult years.

25) The amygdala (also part of the limbic system) creates emotional content for memories, mediating depression, irritability, and hostility/aggression, and governing reaction and responses to fear. The amygdala can be considered as the "watchdog" of the brain.

> The impact of childhood abuse or neglect results in a significantly smaller amygdala, raising the risk for depression, irritability and hostility/aggression; and is also responsible for incorrect emotional "memories," absence of fear conditioning, and an increased chance of psychopathic tendencies.

26) The purpose of the cerebellar vermis is to modulate production and release of neurotransmitters, and has a significant number of receptor sites for stress-related hormones.

> The impact of childhood abuse or neglect results in an increase in potential risk for psychiatric symptoms such as depression, psychosis, hyperactivity, and attention deficits, and in rare cases, psychotic symptoms are possible.

EEG PROFILES OF VARIOUS DISORDERS AND ASSOCIATED PHYSIOLOGY

Below are some basic explanations of EEG and disorders based upon overall brain functioning. A more detailed list of disorders and their association to QEEG appears towards the end of this chapter.

BRAIN TOO FAST

See Diagram 29: Brain Too Fast and Brain Too Slow on page 70.

Anxiety

Usually, excessive, fast waves (beta) occur frontally and spread globally as anxiety levels increase. This pattern is usually interpreted as excessive frontal processing activity, which agrees with the research by LeDoux (1996) and indicates that the cortex typically speeds up mental activity to suppress amygdalic over-arousal, perhaps blocking medial forebrain bundle circuits. Frequently, this pattern may appear as reduced slow-wave amplitudes rather than elevated beta.

Beta dominance in anxiety usually has more beta in the right hemisphere than in the left, indicating an effort by the brain to increase the right frontal area to inhibit limbic activity.

Research indicates that the right frontal region is a key area for inhibiting emotion. Theta is also low in amplitude, but appears higher than alpha on eyes-closed baseline. If beta continues to grow in amplitude on the right, then it often indicates mania or aggressive behavior with raging. In general, the frontal beta is usually indicative of worry. Posterior beta is indicative of rumination. Elevated beta is suggestive of trauma or PTSD, as beta blocks input from the limbic system (input from the limbic system shows up in theta). When we see increases in beta, alpha usually drops out.

Anxiety often creates attentional problems and from a symptomology standpoint looks like ADD and ADHD.

Daniel Amen is a renowned clinician and author who specializes in SPECT scans for diagnostic purposes. He believes (1998) a connection between basal ganglia activity and anxiety exists. Since the dopamine circuit plays a central role in basal ganglia activity, and appears elevated in conditions where the brain is running too fast, there seems to be a connection between an overactive attentional network and high dopamine levels.

The basal ganglia have strong efferent connections with the premotor strip through the ventral anterior thalamus. The basal ganglia also connect up to the cingulate and associational networks through the intralaminar nuclei. These same nuclei receive efferents (axonal fibers) from the motor strip and feed information in a loop back to the basal ganglia. The 10-20 locations of Cz and Pz seem to be important areas of possible influence on the attentional system and the dopamine system. Adjustments to this system may be driving the rest of the cortical system, especially in terms of neuromodualtor activity.

Fibromyalgia

Fibromyalgia looks very similar to anxiety except beta amplitudes increase toward the rear and alpha amplitudes increase toward the front. This phenomenon is often called "the backwards brain." This pattern also shows up in chronic fatigue and other physiological disorders. LORETA maps show this activity to be in the posterior cingulate. Standardized low-resolution brain electromagnetic tomography (sLORETA) is a QEEG method of analyzing the EEG and determining the exact source within the cortex of any group of frequencies.

OCD

A meta-analysis of the literature indicates that the only basic distinction reflected by OCD brains is a bilateral difference in hemispheric speed, although presentations by Leslie Prichep, PhD of NYU include discussions of a common high beta background. There appear to be alpha and theta subtypes of OCD, with the alpha subtype being less responsive to existing medications. Many clinicians report excessive fast-wave activity around Fz and interpret it as an overactive cingulate. The cingulate has been implicated as central in the attentional network with regard to discriminating internal from external stimuli. The discriminator theory of consciousness and

LeDoux's (1996) short-term memory and consciousness theories come into play here. The cingulate may be getting stuck on networks concerned with internal stimuli that are threatening due to increased dopamine activity in the basal ganglia (see Chapter Three), which is in turn driven by the mesolimbic activity. The cingulate also connects the frontal and parietal lobes to the parahippocampal gyrus and the temporal lobe. The basal ganglia loop through the intralaminar nuclei may be locking up the whole system and driven by an overactive amygdala.

The question is, where is the best place to intervene in the loop? Fz and Pz seem to be the best candidates from clinical reports. Cz SMR is used successfully by the Othmers (1994, 2008). In addition, research from UCLA by Jeffery Schwartz (2002) indicates the caudate as a key player. He believes he has isolated a worry circuit within the anterior cingulate that fails to manage internal dialogue related to worry in the appropriate manner.

The only case where it did not appear this way showed up as excessive focal alpha in absolute power at Pz. This makes sense, as focal damage to this area often results in perseveration problems. Pz also has direct connections through the lateral dorsal thalamus to the cingulate and the basal ganglia have efferents running through the interlaminar nuclei to Pz connecting motor functions with associative functions. Sherlin and Congedo (2005) have done research indicating that OCD can appear as deviant beta activity anywhere along the cingulate.

BRAIN TOO SLOW

See Diagram 29: Brain Too Fast and Brain Too Slow on page 70.

Depression

Depression usually appears as central slowing with high-amplitude alpha frontally and centrally. More specifically, alpha dominance in depression is in the left hemisphere. The alpha is usually low frequency in the 8 Hz range, but may also drop down as low as 6 Hz to 7 Hz. The lower frequency may indicate how old and entrenched the depression is. On some equipment, depending on filter settings, this may look like high theta. Alpha is the doorway between the limbic system and the cortex. When alpha is low, the door is usually closed. It is easy to confuse depression with head injury and ADD.

Margret Ayers (personal communication) argued that most ADD is really associated with anoxia, stroke, birth trauma, or head injury, which makes sense from an EEG morphological perspective. Beta may still be dominant in the right hemisphere, locking the depression in place with the older anxiety that generated it. To help distinguish between ADD and depression, we use the TOVA and the Beck Depression Inventory. Slowing in the frontal lobes is classic ADHD. Often we see elevated delta and theta in the frontal areas (however, elevated delta in the frontal areas can be indicative of TBI as well).

Atypical Depression

At this point, it is important to discuss atypical depression or depression with anxiety. From our perspective, all depression begins with anxiety (unless it is a result of physical trauma or chemicals). As the anxiety matures, the beta amplitude increases on the right and depletes neurotransmitter systems as the brain slows. As it slows, alpha amplitude increases and moves to the left, shutting down executive function. This process protects the brain.

During this transitional phase, the symptoms of depression appear with the pre-existing anxiety. As the depression matures, the alpha increases in amplitude and slows in frequency, reducing processing. The beta on the right blocks the process from reversing at a certain point and depression becomes profound. This is why increasing beta on the left helps unblock chronic depression, although increasing alpha to the right in the atypical depression is often better.

The original research done on this model was at Keck Labs at the University of Wisconsin by Richard Davidson (2000). Peter Rosenfeld worked with Elsa Baehr (1997) on research showing that training to correct asymmetry can reduce symptoms of depression. Baehr went on to work with Tom Collura to develop a simplified version of this protocol involving increasing alpha on the right while inhibiting it on the left using powerful inhibits. This and other basic protocols are outlined in Chapter Six.

Diagram 29: Brain Too Fast & Brain Too Slow

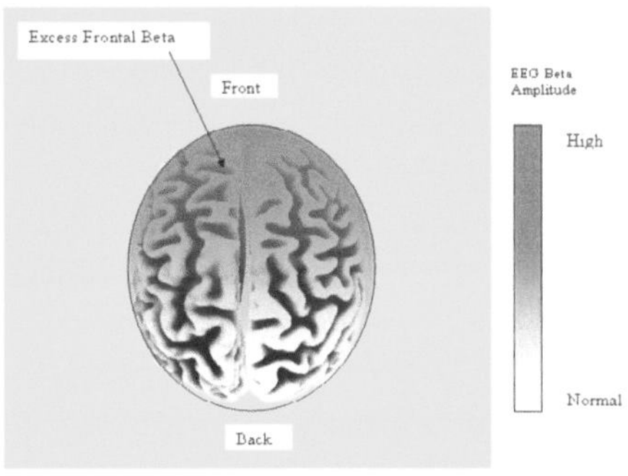

Brain Too Fast 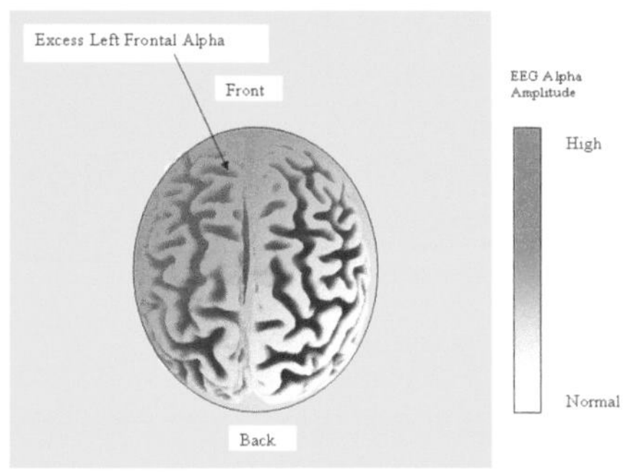   Brain Too Slow

SPECTRAL ANALYSIS

Spectral analysis graphs are available on most EEG equipment systems (see Diagram 30 Spectral Analysis, page 70). They have become very sophisticated and often provide real-time 3D analysis. Using spectral analysis for reviewing the changes in EEG amplitudes over time and in relation to different tasks can be very useful. Lubar (1991, 1999) notes that individuals with ADD have an increase in slow-wave (2-8 Hz) activity when intentionally processing information such as reading and math. Correlating changes reflected in the graph with activities recorded at the same time can reveal hidden dynamics and confirm diagnoses or indicate progress in training.

In conjunction with TOVA scores, progress can be thoroughly documented as clients progressively learn to use the correct circuitry to process information. In fact, on-task spectral analysis graphs probably can provide far more than baseline measures. Presently, QEEGs may include reading and math exercises to clarify attentional and processing problems.

Unfortunately, this kind of analysis may be time consuming and difficult to employ in a clinical setting.

Diagram 30: Spectral Analysis (BrainMaster Technologies)

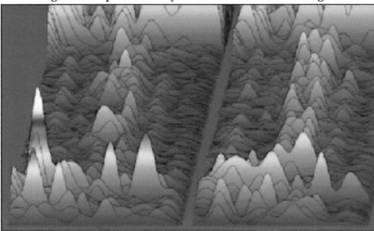

Kirtley Thornton (personal communication), a New Jersey therapist, has spent the last decade developing a clinically friendly testing procedure involving QEEG and a task-based database to evaluate what he considers the three most critical dimensions of cognitive processing: auditory memory, reading memory, and problem solving. His procedure involves much more than spectral analysis.

Brain Maps and Disorders

Brain maps have become progressively more utilized in diagnosis and training strategies in recent years. Their validity for diagnostic purposes is still hotly debated in the field of neurology, but they have been used for a variety of purposes for many years. One has only go to PubMed and use the search term QEEG to uncover the thousands of research papers that have used QEEG. However, and as noted earlier in Chapter Three, recent research continues to bring QEEG brain mapping closer to the realm of diagnostic ability.

QEEG brain mapping use in neurofeedback training is also hotly debated. Since brain mapping is expensive, and not presently covered by all insurance companies, clients often avoid or refuse them. Neurofeedback has been successfully done for decades without them; however, as noted above, we strongly encourage their use, especially for clinicians new to the field. The MiniQ has been specifically developed to allow clinicians new to the field to have access to affordable equipment and clinician friendly database report systems.

Historical Overview of Databases

With few commercially developed databases available, QEEG brain mapping was rarely used in this field before 1995. The primary database in use was NxLink. There was a limited distribution of the Thatcher Lifespan Database through Lexicor, whose Neurosearch 24 amplifiers pioneered the process. Only approximately sixty NxLink databases were sold worldwide at a cost of around twelve thousand dollars each. The NxLink database was then the gold standard and it still is considered so by many. Bill Hudspeth was also developing a database system at this time that provided very elegant coherence analysis within one-Hz bins analysis. Although some differences between the databases existed, there was enough congruence between them to make them useful together. Many were using his system in conjunction with the NxLink system for a more comprehensive analysis.

Around the same time, Barry Sterman and David Kaiser began developing a magnitude database system based on Sterman's work and data from Air Force pilots. Arguably, this is a peak-performance database, as it measures normal EEG in an elite population of mostly fighter pilots. This database looked primarily at magnitude distribution, average amplitude, and eventually a new dimension of analysis, co-modulation, was added. (a quick sentence to discuss/introduce magnitude??)

Later in the decade, Robert Thatcher began to intensively develop his database system into what is presently the most sophisticated database analysis system available. This system provides researchers and clinicians with a huge variety of dimensions for analysis for QEEG. With respect to clinical work in neurofeedback, much of it has limited value. With respect to research, it is a stunning tool that has features for research that have yet to be developed.

The MiniQ system was co-developed by Richard Soutar and Tom Collura at BrainMaster. The concept was to provide a data gathering system for entry-level practitioners who could not afford $15,000 to $20,000 for equipment for a cutting-edge technology with limited clinical development and research behind it. The system collected 12 locations of data in homologous pairs in a sequence of 6 one-minute recordings. BrainMaster provided output data on magnitude, coherence, phase, and other dimensions of analysis, but to date no database system was developed.

Soutar and Demos began developing small reference databases for the system and began offering them in 2005. Presently, the New Mind Database System, developed by Soutar, has developed an expert database system that has been cross-validated with the Neuroguide and NxLink databases as well as the SKIL database with respect to normative magnitude values. Coherence and phase are based on non-normative populations. Dominant frequency is based on published norms in the EEG literature and asymmetry measures based on a combination of clinical data and the work of Richard Davidson. The clinical data are derived from a decade of subject symptom correlations between QEEG and the Beck Depression Inventory. The database has a discriminant output based on expert rules as well as neurological research and MRI research. This provides probability levels for a variety of cognitive and emotional problems. In addition, the database system provides output with protocol recommendations based on the published literature and Z-score location recommendations for Z-score training.

QEEG-guided neurofeedback is likely to be the standard in the future. Until recently, it has been mistakenly seen primarily as a method for deriving protocols. It has not proven to be the best and only valid method for all neurofeedback cases in a clinical setting. Often the best protocols to be used in any given case may run counter to what appears obvious on a brain map. This is simply because the complexity of brain networks demands extensive analysis with respect to intervention. Protocols should be developed based on symptoms, QEEGs, a solid understanding of underlying neurophysiology, and clinical experience. What the QEEG does provide is an invaluable overview of what is going on in the brain and the ability to track changes based on protocol selection. Presently, it is being used in this capacity with other medical and psychological interventions. QEEG provides a roadmap, not the specific directions.

QEEG Analysis Procedures

Generally, data are collected from 5 to 19 locations on the scalp using the 10-20 system for electrode placement. Data are collected from all locations simultaneously or in homologous groups. The data are then displayed in the form of standard EEG tracings and artifacts are identified. These artifacts are usually related to eye blinks, eye movement, and electromyography (EMG). The artifacts are manually removed using a computerized artifacting procedure, and the remaining normative samples of EEG are mathematically knitted together. This process provides a high quality record for analysis.

Minimally, one minute of data is required for a good analysis, but generally two minutes are preferred. In order to achieve this, at least five minutes of recording are required for each task. Recordings to be used for court cases need to be at least 10 minutes in length for each condition. Data are collected separately for eyes-open and eyes-closed analyses and labeled accordingly. It is best to record eyes-closed first to reduce the intrusion of stage one sleep into the record. In the case of MiniQ, data are collected in sequences of homologous pairs or groups to capture coherence information.

Once a good record has been generated, it can be analyzed and used to generate topographic maps showing the intensity and distribution of the various components and single-Hz EEG band frequency. The primary EEG data are broken down using mathematical analyses into component bands of delta, theta, alpha, and beta (and sometimes hi-beta). Other dimensions of analysis utilize these same component divisions. For instance, they will look at beta coherence and alpha coherence separately.

Various combinations are presented by different database systems. Fairly standard dimensions of analysis are magnitude, power, coherence, phase asymmetry, frequency, and comodulation. These dimensions are studied independently (univariate) and together in combination (multivariate) to determine abnormal patterns that may correlate with various disorders.

Discriminants

Analysis of the various dimensions together can yield stereotypical patterns that tend to correlate with various disorders. When one is using statistical analysis or expert rules, these dimensions of analysis can yield valuable information for the clinician or researcher. NxLink provided discriminants for a wide variety of disorders. Although their accuracy seemed impressive in a research setting, most of us who use them in a clinical setting find them very misleading and inaccurate. This situation continues today in most of the research-quality databases.

Jay Gunkleman and many other experts advise against the use of discriminants or at the very least suggest a very cautious consideration of these types of reports. Robert Thatcher emphasizes only using them to confirm an existing diagnosis and only when such a diagnosis is present. He explains that these types of tests are subject to the same potential false positives and false negatives of any lab test and should be used in the same manner.

The New Mind discriminants have been developed with these issues in mind and represent a different category of discriminant. They represent only a probability level that a certain cognitive or emotional problem may be present (rather than a diagnostic category). They are based on MRI and autopsy research from the neurology literature and not just on statistical correlation with *Diagnostic and Statistical Manual of Mental Disorders* (DSM) categories. They are used in conjunction with a cognitive-emotional checklist and are, therefore, only confirmatory in nature. The QEEG configurations are grounded in expert clinical observation. The discriminant is used only for neurofeedback purposes and is not designed for medical or psychological diagnosis.

With these features in place, such a discriminant system can be very accurate and useful for neurofeedback purposes. Pioneering such a system has not been easy and has required us to walk a fine line between advocates and critics of the use of discriminants. The system has proven very successful in its preliminary beta test at Old Vineyard Behavioral Health Hospital and in many clinics across the country. Its present users find it extremely accurate. It is now being cross-correlated with the Minnesota Multiphasic Personality Inventory (MMPI) through research at the University of North Carolina. It is also being correlated with nutritional deficiencies at the renowned Whitaker Clinic at Newport Beach in California. With continued cautious development, discriminant analysis is expected to become the norm in QEEG-guided neurofeedback of the future.

Three factors, in addition to the psychological factors, influence EEG:

1. Biological factors,
2. Social /environmental factors, and
3. Equipment.

Taking good baselines and using general protocols that have been developed to deal with various disorders are often adequate. However, difficult cases like head injury, stroke, and some ADD cases may require a brain map. Overall, maps make training much easier because they provide a clear picture of the EEG dynamics at work. The New Mind Apps brain mapping system makes this position more clear and is explained below.

The International Society for Neurofeedback Research (ISNR) recently published a position paper in the *Journal of Neurotherapy* (Hammond et al., 2004) indicating that although brain maps are not required for neurofeedback, they are preferred. This does not mean they expect everyone to run out and buy $10,000 worth of databases and brain mapping equipment. It does mean, however, that they would prefer qualified practitioners do some form of mapping, if only a MiniQ. (A MiniQ is a standard mapping system that maps at 10 sites: F3 & F4, C3 & C4, P3 & P4, T3 &T4,

and O1 & O2, wheras a full Q measures at 19 sites: Fz, Cz, & Pz; Fp1, & Fp2, F3, & F4, F7 & F8; C3, & C4; T3, & T4, T5 & T6; P3 & P4; and O1 & O2.)

Diagram 31: Early Brain Map from the Nx Link Database, on page 76, presents a typical early brain map. There are representations for absolute power, relative power, asymmetry, and coherence. In each of these categories there are images representing conventional frequency bands of delta, theta, alpha, and beta. These may not always be adequate for analysis; some databases offer one-Hertz breakdowns or "one-Hertz bins," as they are often called. In this case, each image, or map, represents only one frequency.

The absolute power images represent the electrical power in each band of EEG compared to all other individuals in the database. The color coding represents the intensity of the difference between the subject/client and the normative group. In this example, black is normal, and white represents extremely high amounts of power. Light blue represents extremely low power. This power is measured in Z-scores, or units of deviations from the average. The scale at the top of the page ranges from one to three in either a positive or negative direction. Power (magnitude) in QEEG is computed by the formula of voltage squared divided by frequency (V^2/f). This is different from the standard formula of voltage squared divided by resistance (V^2/r). Consequently, many people involved in the electronics side of this business are uncomfortable with this interpretation. The difference is because we are dealing with AC theory in EEG certain assumptions are made regarding resistance and capacitance of the brain, dura matter, and skull. During a conversation with Robert Thatcher, he indicated that the resistance of the brain was very low and fairly consistent, perhaps around 8 Ohms.

The relative power images represent the power in one frequency band compared to all other bands. This measurement is then compared to all other similar measurements of other individuals in the database. In many cases this comparison can be more useful as a measurement because the total power of each person's EEG varies so much. It is often more accurate to look at the differences in each frequency band with regard to the person's own EEG. The proportional relationships between each band within the individual's own EEG offer a more accurate picture of how that person differs from others.

Robert Thatcher warns users of his database system to be extremely careful in using relative power because he feels it greatly distorts the general picture. Over the years, however, it has proven to be critical for clinical assessment when individuals have very high or low power globally. Because of the number of individuals encountered with low power EEG, we have become skeptical of the concept that there is only one distribution in the human EEG. We use three different distributions for analysis in the New Mind Database System.

The asymmetry images are developed using information from the absolute power readings. They tell us the difference in power between the left side and the right side of the brain. Although a person may have lower than average alpha, he or she may still have more alpha on the right than the left, which would be normal.

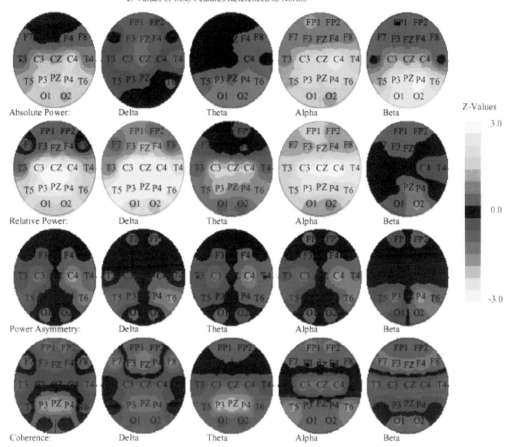

Diagram 31: Early Brain Map from the Nx Link Database

Z-Values of EEG Features Referenced to Norms

The coherence images show the areas of the brain that are communicating with other areas. A well-functioning brain is very flexible. This flexibility is reflected in a fairly high degree of differentiation between sites. Pairs showing a Z-score of -3 would be communicating too little, while pairs showing Z-scores of +3 would probably be communicating too much. However, too much differentiation (or too little) might mean the areas are not working well together at all. Some databases do a better job than others in communicating this ability in images. Consequently, it is better to rely on the numbers. In fact, the numbers often give a clearer picture of what is happening.

Note: In general, with eyes closed, alpha is dominant, followed by theta, delta, and then beta. With eyes closed, alpha is increased and beta is decreased. With eyes open, delta is dominant, followed by theta, alpha, and then beta. The mean dominant frequency of alpha can predict the entire speed of the brain.

SUBCOMPONENT ANALYSIS

The following quick guide is useful in understanding the subcomponent analysis system of the New Mind Maps brain mapping system (see Diagram 32: Sub Component Analysis, below).

- Delta Red is indicative of white matter damage.
- Delta Blue is indicative of too little to no continuity (connectivity).
- Theta Red is indicative of injury to cortex stroke (4-7 red), ADD, or TBI.
- Theta Blue is indicative of lack of emotional connection or lack of memory.
- LoAlpha Red is indicative of metabolic issues, hyperthyroid, or other thyroid problems.
- LoAlpha Blue is indicative of anxiety (in children it can be mylination problems).
- HiAlpha Red is indicative of possible head injury.
- HiAlpha Blue is indicative of anxiety and PTSD.
- LoBeta Red is indicative of anxiety and depression mixed.
- LoBeta Blue is indicative of not blocking information from motor strip, fibromyalgia, or overwhelm from sensory input.
- Beta Red is indicative of worry (15-12 red) insomnia.
- Beta Blue is indicative of cognitive deficit.
- HiBeta Red is indicative of hypervigilance.
- HiBeta Blue is indicative of under-arousal.

Diagram 32: Sub Component Analysis

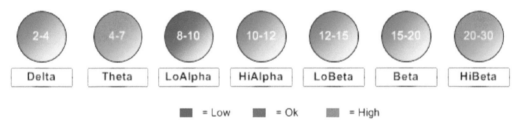

Diagram 33: Discriminants Analysis

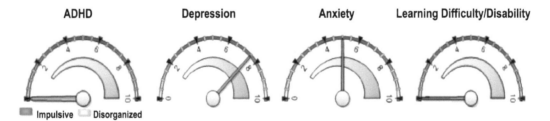

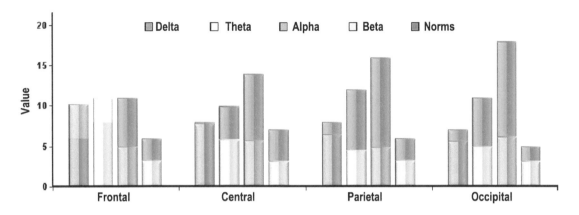

Learning to use brain maps effectively is an art as well as a science and requires considerable one-on-one training with real cases. It is best to take several workshops on the subject and to develop a relationship with someone who has been reading them for a long time. However, even novices can begin to see the patterns in the relative power and asymmetry measures.

The maps of individuals with bipolar disorder change as they shift from one end of the disorder's continuum to the other. Even though most individuals have very stable maps that don't change over time, certain factors can confound their maps. Too little sleep or drugs such as antihistamines can increase theta. A healthy person can shift his or her alpha asymmetry, so alpha increases in the left hemisphere, by thinking of a very sad event, then shift it back to the right by thinking of a happy event. Elsa Baehr used a grad student to demonstrate this in real time at one of her workshops. However, there is a difference between the healthy grad student and a disregulated client. Through effort, the grad student canshift asymmetry whereas a client most likely cannot.

A SUMMARY GUIDE TO ASSIST WITH BRAIN MAP INTERPRETATION[21]

A brain mapping system provides the clinician with several parameters of data to best determine potential problem areas and NFB protocols. Brain maps provide the following:

- a summary of data taken from each measured site

magnitude, coherence, phase, dominant frequency, and asymmetry readings for delta, theta, alpha, and beta (

- Diagram 35: Brain Map from a QEEG Mapping System, page 79)
- a subcomponent analysis for delta, theta, lo-alpha, hi-alpha, lo-beta, beta, and hi-beta (Diagram 32: Sub Component Analysis, page 77)

---

[21] Adapted from: https://newmindmaps.com/

- a discriminant analysis for ADHD, depression, anxiety, and learning disabilities (as shown in Diagram 28: Spectrum Model of Disorders, page 66)
- a cognitive analysis with over 20 categories
- an emotional analysis with 20 categories
- a midline analysis chart (Diagram 34 on page 78)
- suggested supplements
- NFB protocols analysis
- metabolic categories

Diagram 35: Brain Map from a QEEG Mapping System

Magnitude

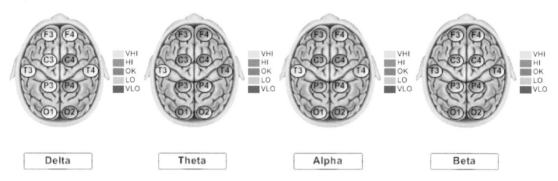

Coherence

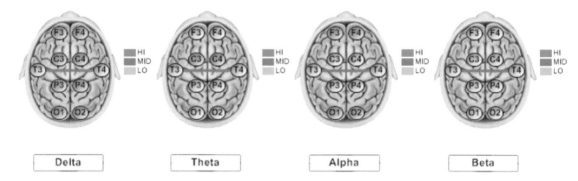

Phase

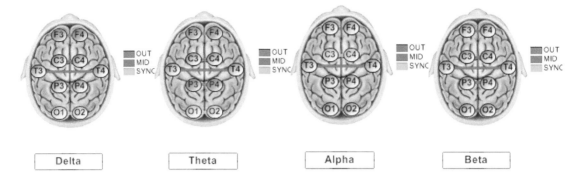

| Delta | Theta | Alpha | Beta |

Dominant Frequency

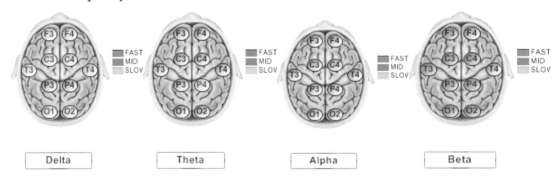

| Delta | Theta | Alpha | Beta |

Asymmetry

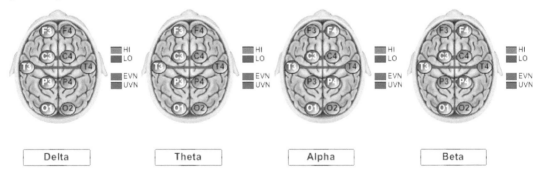

| Delta | Theta | Alpha | Beta |

The following are definitions to assist with understanding how to read and interpret brain maps.

QEEG

Learning to process and read QEEG reports typically takes years of experience, but MiniQ systems such as the *New Mind* Magnitude Analysis System, and those of John Demos and Paul Swingle for example, allow users to obtain a report that is easy to interpret and use, even for those with minimal experience interpreting QEEGs. This allows inexperienced practitioners to immediately begin using QEEG assessment while learning the ins and outs of QEEG-guided neurofeedback; they grow as neurofeedback providers.

The Magnitude Analysis System provides a reference database system that is tailored specifically for clinicians instead of researchers. Instead of using standard deviations, the maps provide simple output indicating whether EEG is high or low in the various dimensions of analysis. The cognitive output automatically flags areas of possible problems based on correlations between map output and MRI research. Emotional output information provides similar information based on MRI research, standard neurology texts, and clinical experience. Clinicians can see at a glance the salient issues likely to be present due to the EEG distribution and are provided an appropriate protocol option.

Magnitude

Magnitude is the most important reading since it is the power of individual brainwaves. Magnitude is used in the New Mind analysis system instead of power because most neurofeedback practitioners work with magnitude; and is also used in the SKIL database (Sterman Kaiser Imaging Labs, Churchville, NY). It is important that practitioners be able to easily refer to their statistics to see the actual microvolt value when an area receives a "high" indication on the map.

Magnitude is the average amplitude over time. The magnitude values in this map are based on a statistical sample in addition to being cross-validated with the major databases. The meaning of high or low magnitudes varies with location and distribution. Learning to interpret their meaning takes considerable experience. The dashboards in this analysis system are designed to help practitioners interpret the map information. These dashboards indicate potential problems that may be present when magnitudes are high or low.

Power vs. Magnitude

A digital analysis of EEG uses fast Fourier transforms (FFT) of the digital data to break down the raw wave forms recorded from the brain into component bands or single-Hertz bins. The various dimension of analysis used in QEEG are derived mathematically from these transforms.

Power is defined as magnitude squared. This definition has generated some argument in the field as to whether power or magnitude is the best measure of analysis. Barry Sterman has argued for years that power distorts the data significantly enough to be a problem in EEG analysis. However, many mathematicians disagree with him that magnitude is the primary measure of clinical analysis. It is very inconvenient to have maps defined in power when training in magnitude. For this purpose, the New Mind database and the Kaiser Sterman database provide magnitude as the centerpiece for EEG analysis. Sterman argues that measures of power may inflate the differences between component bands and distort the representation of the EEG landscape. If magnitudes of theta are derived at $6\mu V$ and beta at $2\mu V$, and then transformed into power, their new values are $36\mu V$ and $4\mu V$ respectively. This mathematical valuation distorts their relationship considerably from 3 to 1 into a relationship of 9 to 1. As long as this type of mistake is not made, however, power is very useful for analysis.

The concern regarding whether there is only one distribution for the human EEG is a major issue that is rarely considered, but should be more carefully researched. E. Roy John (John et al., 1977) addressed this issue through years of research and established that there was only one normative distribution for the human EEG across all cultures. Although this may be true from a purely mathematical perspective, it may not hold up clinically. There is considerable skewness and kurtosis in any given distribution of human EEG (Thatcher, Walker, Biver, North, & Curtin, 2003). This suggests a problem with Gaussianity with respect to the human EEG. Most databases, except New Mind, are log transformed to provide a more Gaussian distribution to generate robust parametrical analysis. This mathematical sleight of hand is perfectly acceptable with respect to many variables, but it may not be okay with human EEG.

Decades of clinical experience with normative databases have revealed a significant population with globally low EEG who function either normally or exceptionally well within the social order. They are by definition abnormal, according to the normative databases, and should have some correlating behavioral problem. Often, however, they do not have correlating problems. Considerable research suggests that there is a naturally occurring low-power subtype in the population. If this situation is the case, then the database would be invalid with respect to such persons' evaluations—perhaps even unethical. In fact, there is also a high-power subtype as well. These subtypes can be conveniently ignored by treating them as outliers and eliminating them on statistical principle from the Gaussian definition. The New Mind database utilizes three overlapping distributions at present to avoid this problem and may use more in the future.

Phase

Phase is meaningful mostly in relationship to coherence measures. Low phase means the two locations are working in synchrony. High phase means they are out of step. For example, if alpha coherence is high in the frontal region and phase is very low, then it is likely that you will have high-amplitude synchronous alpha that is locked in place. This means the frontal lobes are very much in a state of neutral. This state is commonly found in people meditating.

Phase and coherence may be difficult to understand for individuals just learning about mapping. Their relevance with respect to determining protocols for neurofeedback is still not very clear. Training for coherence and phase are very new areas of activity, and little research has been presented on the topic. (If phase is low and coherence is high, then there is a very high level of very synchronous waves; if phase is high and coherence is low, then the brainwaves and the areas they represent are out of synch).

Coherence

Coherence tells us about the brain's efficiency (or lack of efficiency) and is valid between homologous sites, i.e., P3 & P4, F3 & F4, etc., or through inter-hemisphere sites. Coherence is how much one part of the brain is talking to another part. If areas have high coherence, they are over-communicating (like a traffic jam). If they have low coherence, they are under-communicating. In both cases plasticity and function suffer. For instance, high or low coherence between F3 and F4 likely indicates a problem in the short-term memory networks of the frontal lobes.

The more disordered the brain, the more extreme its coherence readings. In more technical terms, coherence is how consistent the phase relationship is between two locations. Many maps provide coherence readings between regions with little functional connectivity. The New Mind mapping system provides coherence readings only between locations that have strong functional connectivity, which is likely clinically meaningful.

When the waxing and waning of the EEG in two locations are compared, there is usually a difference in the timing of the rise and fall of their amplitudes. One signal leads or lags the other with respect to timing. The difference between the two is described through vector analysis and results in comparisons made in terms of degrees. Signals may lead or lag each other by 0 degrees, 90 degrees, or 180 degrees. If they are 180 degrees out of phase, then one signal is at its peak when the other is at its trough. If they consistently lead or lag each other by the same degree over a period of time, they are said to be coherent. This is measure in terms of correlational statistics and may be reported as a Pearson correlation co-efficient.

Problems with Coherence

The extensive use of a variable does not qualify its legitimacy. Often research indicates that a variable has flaws and should be further developed to achieve better measurement. This situation has been the case with the variable of coherence. Coherence has proven to be of limited use clinically and has possibly confounded a great deal of research due to its flaws as a concept and a unit of measurement. Roberto Pascual-Marque, who developed LORETA imaging, has characterized it as a two-dimensional correlate that indicates only a statistical relationship and not necessarily a physical relationship. This condition is partly because a large component is composed of noise from volume conduction and thalamic input may confound the validity of the connectivity measure. David Kaiser, who developed the SKIL database with Barry Sterman, has characterized coherence as a one-dimensional measure, but notes it does have value in conjunction with other measures such as comodulation. Many of the pathways indicated on coherence maps do not exist at the anatomical level, such as between P3 and F4. With this in mind, it is difficult to decide what exactly is being measured other than coincidental correlation. Kaiser and Gunkleman, citing Nunez and other neurophysicists recommend that coherence is more accurate when first transformed using Laplacian analysis. Robert Thatcher, however, makes strong mathematical arguments to the contrary and has broad support from many mathematicians.

The original NxLink database, first developed and marketed by E. Roy John, used homologous sites to generate coherence maps. These were considered the most robust connections with clear clinical relevance. For this reason, we have continued with that tradition in the New Mind MiniQ database. These connections tend to be good proxy measures of general connectivity levels and provide a sufficient sample of coherence for present neurofeedback purposes.

There are those who are using coherence measures for the purposes of training coherence with neurofeedback. Many practitioners have noted that coherence training is fraught with peril and many abreactions and should be approached cautiously with expert guidance. The Z-score training developed by Mark Smith for BrainMaster Technologies appears to have diminished this risk to the point where coherence training is safe for almost anyone. The question still remains, however, what exactly clinicians are training when they train coherence. They may be training power with a proxy two-dimensional correlation measure or they may be training with some rudimentary form of connectivity. Still, clinical reports indicate that coherence training is powerful and has impact on clients when other approaches fail. The bottom line is that there are no studies to evaluate it either way.

Functional vs. Effective Connectivity: The Default Mode

It is clear that the value of QEEG is that it records the temporal dynamics of the idling brain. This information is valuable, as recent research indicates this idling state, now known as the default mode, tells a great deal about the functional connectivity of any given brain. "Functional connectivity" is a term emerging in the neuroimaging sciences that describes the healthy functioning of the brain in terms of normal connections. Are all the hubs and nodes of the brain properly connected and operating in normal range? This condition can be best determined by recording brains "at rest." In this state, people are typically engaged in the routine busywork of the brain organized around keeping their autobiographical selves intact and justified. For highly social animals like human beings, this process is critical for survival. Human beings do it constantly as if their lives depended on it, because their lives do depend on it. A healthy brain has a characteristic resting pattern; deviations from this pattern suggest that functional problems may exist.

"Effective connectivity," on the other hand, tells how well areas communicate while given some task. This type of dynamic measurement is more reflected in task-based databases that involve reading or math such as the one developed by Kirkley Thornton (2000). This subject has been a more traditional area of interest in MRI research. Recently, the research community has recognized that by combining the temporal resolution of QEEG with the spatial resolution of MRI, they can obtain much more comprehensive data.

Unfortunately for clinicians, MRI equipment costs millions to purchase and maintain. However, modern QEEG is an excellent and inexpensive modality of neuroimaging that draws evaluative power from its cross-correlation with MRI in the research domain. It is more than enough because of the spatial resolution limitations of neurofeedback. Interestingly, sLORETA may provide a more suitable platform in the future for medical and pharmacological applications.

Dominant Frequency

Dominant frequency is probably the third most important measure. This measure indicates whether the frequency in a specific component band has slowed down or sped up. For instance, alpha in a healthy person should average between 9.5 and 10.5 Hz. If the dominant alpha frequency drops below 9.5 Hz, then most likely a problem exists. Slowed alpha is often an indicator of depression or physical problems, such as hypothyroid. In this case the modal frequency would be low and show more 8-10 Hz in the subcomponent analysis.

Asymmetry

Asymmetry is second most important in determining if the brain is working properly. For example, increased theta in right front is indicative of impulsivity, while increased theta in left front is indicative of disorganization. When delta is predominantly high on the right, it is indicative of emotional issues; when delta is predominantly high on the left, it is indicative of cognitive issues. There has been considerable research done by Richard Davidson (1995, 2000) regarding EEG asymmetry and its relationship to mood and anxiety. Most databases today do not reflect this research very well, but clinicians find it an important source of information.

This analysis system has been set up so that you can easily read the asymmetries present and compare them to problems your client is reporting. More alpha on the left than the right side usually indicates depression. More beta on the right side than the left usually indicates anxiety. If theta is unusually high and dominates on the left side, it usually indicates a problem with organization. When theta dominates on the right side, it usually indicates a problem with impulsivity.

Comodulation

David Kaiser and Barry Sterman did not have coherence measures in their database system, but saw the need for their own connectivity measures. They have been aware of the many flaws of coherence and have developed an alternative connectivity measure known as comodulation. This measure looks at the covariation of magnitude between two sites and has proven very useful in discriminating clinical problems. It clearly has a valuable future as a dimension of EEG evaluation, but at present is not widely used.

LORETA

This method of EEG analysis was first thought to be the holy grail of QEEG. It soon proved to be another interesting, but flawed, clinical tool for evaluation. Recent improvements have increased its accuracy and value. As soon as we understand connectivity better, it may prove to be one of the best estimates of connectivity available for clinical work. At present, however, connectivity is poorly understood by neuroscience.

SUBCOMPONENT ANALYSIS - SINGLE-HERTZ BINS

The better research quality database systems like Neuroguide usually include a page showing single-Hertz bins. This information provides a topographical distribution analysis for each frequency band and assists in identifying exactly which frequency in a component band is most abnormal as well as what location where it is most dominant. It is very useful for setting filter parameters for training. For instance, if alpha is high in magnitude and needs to be trained down, the practitioner needs to know whether it is high-frequency alpha, low-frequency alpha, or the whole component band. Single-Hertz bins can provide that information by showing that it is only the 8-10 Hz band that is high and that it is high in the frontal region. Unfortunately, practitioners may find that 8-10 Hz alpha is high frontally, but 10-12 Hz alpha is high in the posterior region. This information results in a picture that is confusing, so that it tends to overwhelm beginners—often, even the more advanced map reader. In addition, single-Hertz bins often looks different with respect to magnitude and symmetry from the component band analysis.

In the New Mind database system, the single-Hertz bin concept is adjusted to make it more clinically friendly. The single-Hertz bins are grouped into small component bands that have proven consistently to be correlated with various disorders or behavioral and cognitive features. The distinctions are then based not on some arbitrary mathematical determinant, but on extensive clinical experience. The dominant frequency is presented as the most salient with respect to overall distribution and the key frequency in a given single-Hertz range. The result is an easy-to-understand bird's-eye view of the general lay of the land with respect to frequency distribution.

SUMMARIZATION OF KEY POINTS IN READING BRAIN MAPS

Delta

Delta is generated from the brain stem resonances and the cerebellum. Delta measures do not give clear indications for diagnostics. Parietal delta (P4) affects association and cortex/processing. A delta deficit is indicative of problems with working memory. Arrhythmic delta is normal, while rhythmic delta may indicate pathology. A high delta/beta ratio may indicate slowing (for example eyes-closed delta is 15 and eyes-closed beta is 5). Increased global delta may indicate cognitive decline with age (delta, theta, and alpha start to slow). Table 4 shows delta wave indicators below.

Table 4: Delta Wave Indicators

Area	Indicator	Indicator	Indicator	Indicator	Indicator
Frontal	TBI	LD	Dementia	Parkinson's	Decreased delta may indicate short-term memory problems
Temporal	TBI	Language processing problems			Short-term memory problems
Global	TBI				Emotional processing problems /ADHD / list acquisition problems
Posterior		LD			

Theta

Theta issues develop from the anterior cingulate input into the cortex. Theta is driven by the limbic system and is involved with memory searching, network linking, and emotional valence. Theta emerges from the hippocampal loop (the septal hippocampal circuits/limbic system). Theta issues may develop from input from the anterior cingulate into the cortex or may indicate focal activation problems in the cortex. Generally, when there is increased theta, there may be increases in delta and alpha (all slower waves). Havng increased theta and beta is like driving with the brakes on (the brain does not run smoothly).

A theta/beta ratio greater than 3:1 constitutes a slow-wave disorder. The normal theta/beta ratio is 2:1 (i.e., theta 8.7 over beta 11.07 = .79 or too much beta). The largest theta/beta ratios are found at Cz or Fz; the smallest theta/beta ratios are found in the temporal lobes. The normal theta/beta ratio at Cz is 1.6:1, and at Fpz is 1.5:1. A high theta/beta ratio is a signature of ADHD (i.e., 2.5:1). Children with ADHD often show a 3:1 ratio. Table 5 on page 87 shows theta wave indicators.

Table 5: Theta Wave Indicators

Area	Indicator	Indicator	Indicator	Indicator	Indicator
Frontal	ADHD / ADD Anxiety	Impulsiveness/ Impulse control D/O / lack of inhibitory control (When theta is higher on the right front and right hemisphere)	Foggy headed /LD (Unable to grasp concepts, ideas, information)	Emotional: PTSD / Depression / Overwhelmed / Emotions shut down.	Disorganization (when theta is higher on the left front and left hemisphere).
Temporal			Language processing problems Short-term memory problems	Emotional processing problems	
Global		Decreased delta globally may indicate a person is low energy (especially when alpha is high)		Emotional processing problems	Trouble with accessing emotional information. Retrieval problems.
Posterior	Pain and anxiety. Decreased theta may indicate attentional problems.	OCD / Perseveration (hard time letting go).	LD Reading comprehension problems.		

Alpha

Alpha is generated from resonance between the thalamus and the cortex. The brain idles in alpha, and constantly shifts up into beta and down into theta. The traumatized brain idles too fast (in the beta direction), or too slowly (in the theta direction). If excessive alpha coherence is present, the brain may be locked up in alpha and be hard to speed up or slow down. Low alpha may be indicative of anxiety, PTSD, or short-term memory impairment. (Low alpha increases cortisol in the brain, which affects the hippocampus and thus short-term memory). Alpha should be higher in the right hemisphere than in the left hemisphere. Alpha asymmetry and locally increased alpha are indicative of depression. With an eyes-closed map, the normal dominant frequency should be alpha. When the dominant frequency is at 11-12 Hz, it is faster than normal; slower than normal from 8-9 Hz and when 9.5-10.5 Hz it is considered normal. Slow (or low) alpha can be indicative of metabolic problems, toxin-related issues, bipolar disorder/depression, and substance abuse (i.e., marijuana use/abuse). Increased fast alpha in the posterior may indicate emotional rumination. Table 6, on page 88, shows alpha wave indicators.

Table 6: Alpha Wave Indicators

Area	Indicator	Indicator	Indicator	Indicator
Frontal	Depression (alpha asymmetry with more alpha on the left than on the right). Lack of motivation.	Decreased alpha is indicative of impulsivity, being controlled by anxiety, feeling overwhelmed, and impulsivity with explosiveness.	ADD Attentional problems.	Pain and anxiety.
Global	Increased alpha on the left may indicate emotional shutdown.	Depression Metabolic issues Substance abuse.	Parkinson's may include alpha slowing.	Person's energy level is low (especially when delta is low).
Posterior	Depression, passivity, and avoidant personality.	Trauma PTSD.		Fibromyalgia (decreased alpha).

Beta

Beta is generated from resonances within the cortex. Beta should be higher on the left than on the right. Increased beta asymmetry in the right hemisphere is indicative of anxiety. Global elevated beta on the right hemisphere is generally indicative of anxiety (look at magnitude and asymmetry). Increased beta in the left frontal area blocks amygdala input. Beta hyper-coherence may indicate anxiety, panic attacks, and test anxiety. Panic attacks can look like full-body seizures—especially when there are sensory integration problems.

Dominant frequency beta may indicate that there is excess norepinephrine. Increased beta alone is often indicative of withdrawal from social interaction (when theta and alpha are lower). Increased beta at Fp2 and F3 simultaneously can be indicative of the patient hiding all feelings and emotions (flat affect may be seen). Increased beta and decreased alpha in frontalis is indicative of agitation, being controlled by anxiety, feeling overwhelmed, and impulsivity with explosivenessTable 7 on page 89 shows beta wave indicators.

Table 7: Beta Wave Indicators

Area	Indicator	Indicator	Indicator	Indicator	Indicator
Frontal	Anxiety Impulsivity (being controlled by anxiety and feeling overwhelmed), and impulsivity with explosiveness. Mood shifts.	Pain	Emotional Hyper-vigilance and controlling, passive, and/or avoidant personality Insomnia Person hides all feelings and emotions (flat affect may be seen).	Fear (increased frontal beta) Aggression (decreased frontal beta)	Increased beta in frontal areas and in the right hemisphere (the brain is running too fast) may indicate anxiety, OCD, mania, and worry.
Temporal	TBI			Anger Irritability	
Global	Anxiety ADD Insomnia (insomnia often reveals LoBeta/Beta at 5.1/4.5).	Insomnia Muscle tension Headaches	Self-regulation problems.		OCD
Posterior	Anxiety disorder(s) Rumination.	Fibromyalgia	Rumination Trauma.		OCD Rumination.

EEG CORRELATES OF DISORDERS

QEEG is not considered a diagnostic tool at this time; however, the QEEG may indicate and or validate a particular disorder or concern. Certain QEEG profiles may be indicative of one or more disorders.

Anger, Fear, Irritability, and Aggression

Right hemisphere frontal activity is often associated with the amygdala's response to fear. Aggressive patients have excessive slow waves in the frontal area; they can't control the fear, so they act out. ADD and anxiety may indicate that the patient can be explosive. Patients with irritability and anger usually have temporal lobe problems. The patient may be over-aroused.

Anxiety

Anxiety results from elevated amygdala action. The activity travels to the thalamus and inputs into the medial frontal cortex. The hypothalamus controls hunger, thirst, sex drive, and body temperature. Anxiety is the brain's first line of defense. Anxiety is associated with too much fast-wave (beta) activity in the right frontal area. Anxiety can have a global impact through the amygdala and RAS enhancement of norepinephrine. Increased activity in the amygdala often displays increased beta at Fp1 and Fp2. Increased beta activity in the frontal area blocks worry and anxiety. Anxiety problems lead to memory and retention problems.

ADD/ADHD

Often, ADD presents as slowing of the brain's electrcal activity. ADHD shows increased frontal theta in the left and right hemispheres (short-term memory). Learning disabilities and ADHD may indicate white matter problems..

Bipolar Disorder

Bipolar disorder usually reveals increased beta in the right hemisphere and frontal beta (during the manic phase). During the depressive cycle, there is usually low frequency alpha in the frontal area.

Cognitive Concerns

Temporal lobe theta may indicate language and memory processing problems. Temporal lobe delta may also indicate language and memory processing problems, or if it is coming from the insula just above the temporal lobes, it may indicate integration problems between the cortex and the peripheral nervous system. Emotional valence is also affected by abnormalities of the temporal lobes.

Depression

When patients become depressed, they have exhausted their systems through being anxious all the time. The left frontal area slows down and depression sets in. Depression usually reveals increased alpha on the left side and may often be displayed as increased global alpha, especially in the midbrain (emotion). Depression can look exactly like ADHD in children. When patients are angry, bargain, whine, and are hyperactive, it may be depression, not ADHD.

Physical Pain

High amplitude non-rhythmic theta and delta bursts are often seen with migraine headaches. They are usually combined with excessive beta in the cingulate, as is high blood pressure. Pain is often associated with excessive activity in the cingulate, especially the anterior cingulate. Sterman and Kaiser have identified a region around the insula, which is often especially active in pain, that can often be trained to assist in pain reduction.

Trauma and PTSD

The patterns associated with PTSD vary and a precise distribution has not emerged. However, many key features often appear present. PTSD reveals increased posterior beta, alpha deficit, and high frontal coherence. When a patient experiences fear, right-side beta increases to shut down panic. The patient will pull back more. PTSD often reveals increased 16-19 beta globally. The frontal area lights up with beta and looks like severe insomnia. When patients are in a chronic state of hyperarousal, the brain exhausts or depletes the neurotransmitters and omega 3 (60% of the brain is fat, of which 25% is omega 3), which means the brain is often overloaded with omega 6 and omega 9. The amygdala is blocked when there is excessive beta activity. Increased 13-15 beta in the frontal lobes blocks emotional information (emotions are kept at bay).

The "Normative Problem"

A well-known editor for some of the major texts on neurofeedback confessed a serious concern about the concept of "normalcy." E. Roy John and Leslie Prichep addressed this issue in their original research, but many experts in sociology and psychology are not satisfied with their treatment.

A whole book could be written on this topic, but we will attempt to be concise here. To make things worse, the preliminary screening test data for NxLink has never actually been published. Testing for other databases is quite flawed as well. Much of the screening for the existing databases has provided valuable data and has narrowed the population in the direction of psychological "normalcy," but may prove to be very insufficient in the long term. Taking a large population sample, randomly selecting from it, and then cross-correlating the EEG distributions with known psychological and sociological measures is proposed. This process would be a more honest appraisal of the total potential variance in the EEG of the human population. It is for these purposes that an internet-based QEEG system for New Mind has been set up. Presently, several universities are participating in the project. No doubt political and economic issues will drive many critical arguments—thinly veiled as scientific—against the project, but then again, science has always been highly political and economically driven.

Miscellaneous Diagnostics
- Lack of blood flow to the brain increases delta and theta waves, and to a lesser degree alpha waves.
- Damage to focal areas results in stereotypical deficits that have been consistently noted in neurology. Slow-wave activity in these areas may have similar effects.
- Focal damage to the central parietal region in the area of the posterior cingulate (Pz) typically results in perseveration.
- Frontal circuits include three basic executive circuits. Increased frontal (Fz) beta indicates the brain being overactive, which affects attention and decision making. Excessive delta and theta have a slowing effect, and the brain is underactive.
- The anterior cingulate (Fz) is the gateway to dorsal lateral circuits. The anterior cingulate processes attention and decision making.
- At Cz with eyes-closed and along the other midline sites (Fpz, Fz, Pz, Oz) the norm is that alpha is dominant at approximately 14 uV, theta 10 uV, delta 8 uV, and beta 7 uV.

Lesion Research

Below are listed behavioral correlates of focal lesions from the neurological literature. High levels of theta in the regions listed often have a similar impact.

Left Hemisphere

Fp1   Orbito frontal circuit—socially cavalier

F3   Dorsolateral circuit—depression, short-term memory difficulty, word retrieval problems, and problem-solving difficulty (Wisconsin Card Sort)

F7   Word retrieval problems, recall difficulties, difficulty filtering environment, and irritability

Temporal

T3   Self-deprecation, episodic memory problems, especially event sequencing, difficulties with verbal-emotional understanding, reading difficulties

T5   Difficulty making sense of events, problems understanding meaning, problems understanding what is read

Parietal

P3   Memory, organization, digit span problems

Beta Correlates

The same research indicates behavioral correlates of excess beta activity in the areas listed below.

Fp1   Dislike novelty, over-focus on structure and predictability

F3   Obsessional thinking

T3   Cortical irritability

T5   Constant confusion/questioning

P3   Excessive thinking and worrying

Right Hemisphere

Fp2   Emotional impulsivity, poor social awareness, socially inappropriate behavior, edginess and anxiety, over-talkativeness

F4   Poor organization of dialogue, poor use of analogy and irony, impolite discourse

F8   Too little prosody

Temporal

T4   Anger, sadness, aggression, emotional tonality problems, voice tonality problems

REVIEW QUESTIONS

1) What are the some of the impacts of trauma on the brain?

2) What are the differences between "brain too slow" and "brain too fast?"

3) Is QEEG widely accepted within the fields of NFB or neurology? Why or why not?

4) How are asymmetry measures useful to the clinician?

5) What is magnitude and how does it differ from power?

6) What is coherence and what are some of the problems associated with its interpretation?

7) What are single-Hertz bins?

8) What are the four basic brainwave frequency ranges? What are two indicators of disorders that might be apparent from each range?

Often new practitioners buy equipment and take workshops on how to use it, but find they are lost when they return to their own practices. Before hooking up clients, it is crucial to thoroughly learn how the equipment works and to train with a clinician/mentor who has experience with the same equipment. The nuances of the equipment and how it performs in a clinical setting will emerge.

At the very least, you should begin practicing on yourself. This method is a good way to explore the equipment and try different protocols to see how they feel subjectively. This experience is immensely helpful in understanding how clients respond to training and to help identify progress indicators.

The following contains the information practitioners should minimally understand.

BASIC ELECTRONICS THEORY

Most practitioners coming into the field know little about electronics theory. Since NFB deals with electro-magnetism from the brain and uses electronic equipment to evaluate it, practitioners must know some of this basic theory to save time, confusion, and frustration.

Voltage (volts): The amount of electrical potential between two locations with different electrical charges is measured in volts. Usually the difference is measured between ground and active electrodes. EEG is read in microvolts (μV). It is the most common unit discussed in neurofeedback. For example, when a client's alpha is 30 microvolts, the alpha is very high and needs to be trained down.

Amperage (amps): The flow of electrical energy is usually defined in terms of fluid dynamics. The stream of electricity flowing between two locations has a rate of flow. The material/energy flowing is electrons. The rate of flow of electrons determines the current, which is measured in terms of amperage or amps. This term is not frequently discussed in EEG.

 Resistance (Ohms): This is the resistance to the flow of current. Some elements conduct electricity more readily than others. Those that have few free electrons, such as the scalp, conduct electricity less readily than copper wire, etc. Resistance is measured in terms of heat with a unit called *Ohms*. The input to EEG equipment at the ends of the electrode is measured in a form of resistance known as impedance. Equipment with very high impedance levels usually gets a better EEG signal with less prep work on the scalp.

Ohm's Law ($E = I{\times}R$), where resistance (Ohms) is resistance to the flow of energy (amps).

Ohm's Law is also depicted as

$$V = R{\times}I,$$

$$I = {}^{V}\!/_{R},$$

$$\text{and } R = {}^{V}\!/_{I}$$

These are all ways that the formula for voltage is computed using resistance and current, as is shown in Table 8: Electronics Terms, below.

Table 8: Electronics Terms

Quantity	Symbol	Unit	Sign
Voltage	V or E (energy)	Volt	V (amplitude in EEG)
Current	I	Ampere (amp)	A
Resistance	R	Ohm	O
Power	P	Watt	W

RESISTANCE TO AC = IMPEDANCE / RESISTANCE TO DC = RESISTANCE

Power (watts): Power refers to the actual amount of energy available in the electrical current. This energy may have been originally in the form of water power, diesel fuel, or chemical energy such as batteries or cells. Such energy is transformed into electrical energy through various processes.

Power can be represented mathematically:

$$P = \frac{V^2}{R}$$

where P is power, V is voltage, and R is resistance.

The brain puts out about 30 watts of power and burns about 50% of the body's glucose to do this. Brain maps usually report EEG in terms of power rather than microvolts, which is confusing because most of the statistics on neurofeedback are reported in microvolts. Fortunately, some QEEG database makers are beginning to provide information in microvolts.

Current: There are two kinds of current: direct current (DC) and alternating current (AC). DC flows continuously in one direction. AC flows first in one direction and then in the opposite direction. AC current is the kind you find in the household socket. EEG is originated by DC current in the cells, but emerges as AC current. The EEG microvolt readings obtained on equipment are usually based on peak-to-peak current changes.

Impedance: AC current behaves differently than DC current and requires a special unit of resistance called impedance. Impedance in AC is a unit of resistance and flow of AC. High impedance is desired on equipment input in the mega-Ohm range. Resistance between the scalp and the electrode should be low—10 k Ohms or less. To accomplish this, we buy expensive equipment and scrub the scalp with a abrasive preparation such as Nuprep®.

Capacitance (microfarads, mfd): A capacitor is a component that stores electricity and allows only AC current to pass through it. It is basically two conductors with a resistance in between. It is a relationship that occurs naturally in the world quite frequently. Cell walls act like capacitors and so do electrical wires that are used to hook up clients. Frequently you have to touch wires to drain off an electrical charge that builds up in the wires and distorts your readings. Some clients, during cold dry weather, will give practitioners a mild electrostatic shock when touched, which will end troublesome readings.

Phase: Phase is about the relationship between two AC currents or two electromagnetic wave forms. EEG waves are electromagnetic waveforms that move from positive to negative voltage. Two waveforms may resonate or cancel based on how much they shift from positive to negative at the same time. If two wave forms shift from positive to negative at exactly the same rate, they are in phase. Two wave forms that shift at the opposite rate are out of phase. Diagram 36: Phase Waves, below, shows examples of in-phase and out-of-phase signals. Areas of the brain that emit consistently in-phase signals are doing so because they are communicating and processing the same information. Consequently, they are referred to as coupled.

Diagram 36: Phase Waves

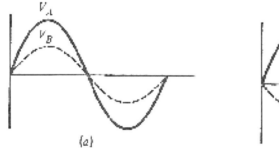 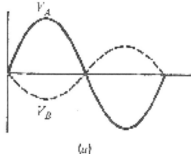

In-phase waves   Out-of-phase waves

COMMON MODE REJECTION

The common-mode rejection ratio (CMRR) of a differential amplifier (or other device) measures the tendency of the device to reject input signals common to both input leads. A high CMRR is important in applications where the signal of interest is represented by a small voltage fluctuation superimposed on a (possibly large) voltage offset (voltage offset may have no meaning to most people), or when relevant information is contained in the voltage difference between two signals. An example is audio transmission over balanced lines.

CMRR is often important in reducing noise on transmission lines. In the case of EEG, artifact may occur from a variety of sources: EMG, blinking, outside electrical interference, etc. For example, when measuring, make it a common-mode voltage signal. The CMRR of the measurement instrument determines the attenuation (reduction of background noise) applied to the offset or noise. In short, common mode rejection does the following:

27) detects the difference between the active and reference electrode, then

28) subtracts the difference between active and reference, then

29) rejects unwanted signals common to both amplifier inputs

FAST FOURIER TRANSFORM

Fast Fourier transform (FFT) is the mathematical method of calculating the frequency composition of a wave. A good metaphor for this is the prism. When held up to sunlight, a prism breaks light down into a rainbow spectrum of colored light bands. These are the light frequencies that, when combined, make up white light. Like a prism, FFT analysis breaks up the composite EEG into its individual frequency components, decoding the raw wave forms into individual frequencies.

HOW EQUIPMENT WORKS

Electrodes attached to the head must pick up an electrical signal (waveforms) that is highly attenuated. Voltages beneath the skull are in the millivolt (mV) range, but voltages at the surface of the scalp are in the microvolt range (μV) (see Diagram 37: Microvolt Ranges and Wavelengths, below). This is because the skull has a great deal of resistance and is not a good conductor of electricity, below. To help make a good connection with the scalp, apply electrode paste so that electrons can flow easily from scalp to electrode. If they do not, then the waveforms are distorted.

Diagram 37: Microvolt Ranges and Wavelengths

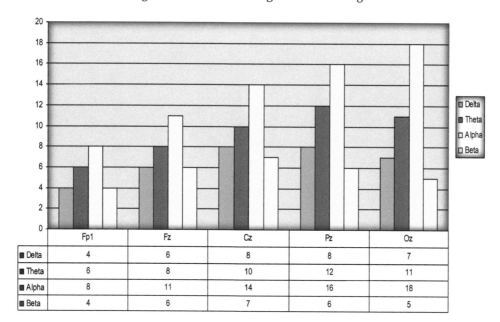

	Fp1	Fz	Cz	Pz	Oz
■ Delta	4	6	8	8	7
■ Theta	6	8	10	12	11
■ Alpha	8	11	14	16	18
■ Beta	4	6	7	6	5

Since microvolts are too small to measure easily, a special type of amplifier is used to help increase the amplitude of the waveform so the computer can use it. This amplifier is also able to reject undesired electrical signals. When picking up a signal in microvolts, it is also easy to pick up tiny signals from other sources since electricity is everywhere at this voltage level. A device known as a differential amplifier employing common mode rejection is used. Diagram 38: Differential Amplifier, below shows a diagram of such a device. It has two inputs for EEG signals and a third reference input. Any signals that are out of phase with the EEG signals are cancelled and only the EEG signals pass through the amplifier. They are made larger in amplitude through an initial stage of pre-amplification so that other stages of amplifiers can increase them more. Eventually they are large enough to be digitized and passed on to the computer for useto be used for NFB feedback.

Before the amplified EEG signals reach the screen, they are often broken down into their respective frequency ranges. This way, the raw EEG or a filtered version that shows delta, theta, alpha, and beta (lo-beta, beta, and hi-beta) can be viewed. The filters used for this process are either physical components called analogue filters, or virtual components called fast Fourier transforms.

The analogue filters give real-time results, while there is a very slight delay in fast Fourier. This delay happens because the equipment must do ongoing calculations with the signal information in order to break it down into fundamental components and reconstruct it into frequency bands. There are arguments regarding the effects of such a delay. The use of "digital" filters has enhanced the speed of almost all modern equipment. In fact, Margaret Ayers marketed equipment that theoretically has no digital delay.

Diagram 38: Differential Amplifier

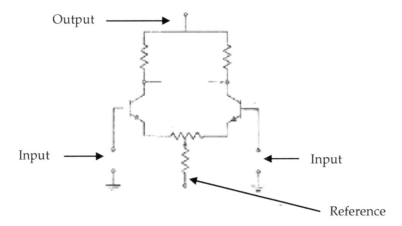

With EEG, there are various filters that can or may be applied. Most commonly we hear about low-pass filters and high-pass filters.

Low-pass Filter: A low-pass filter is a filter that allows lower frequency signals to pass but attenuates (reduces the amplitude of) signals with frequencies higher than the designated cutoff frequency. The actual amount of attenuation for each frequency varies from filter to filter. When used in audio applications, such a filter is sometimes called a high-cut filter or treble-cut filter.

The concept of a low-pass filter exists in many different forms, including electronic circuits (like a hiss filter used in audio). Low-pass filters play the same role in signal processing that moving averages do in some other fields, such as finance. Both tools provide a smoother form of a signal by removing the short-term oscillations, leaving only the long-term trend. Low-pass filters can be used to block out artifact from muscle tension (EMG) and 60 Hz noise from a poor ground.

High-pass Filter: High-pass filters decrease artifact. A high-pass filter is a filter that passes high frequencies well, but attenuates (reduces the amplitude of) frequencies lower than the cutoff frequency. The actual amount of attenuation for each frequency varies from filter to filter. Such a filter is sometimes called a low-cut filter; the terms *bass-cut filter* or *rumble filter* are also used in audio applications. A high-pass filter is the opposite of a low-pass filter. High-pass filters can be used to block out eye blink, eye movement, and other low frequency artifacts. A band-pass filter is a combination high-pass and low-pass filter.

DIFFERENCES IN EQUIPMENT

EEG iinstruments are designed differently. Some instruments have two reference leads and a ground and others have only one reference lead and a ground. Some instruments have two or four EEG amplifiers and others have only one. With four amplifiers, four EEGs can be run at once and train or monitor several locations at once. This method can have tremendous advantages.

Some equipment has raw EEG displays and other equipment does not. Since brainwave morphology can supply important information, the latter can be a serious drawback. Some equipment supplies only dichotomous feedback while other devices supply continuous feedback or both. Some have good graphics and others have limited but higher quality graphics.

How and what information is displayed is crucial. It is often nice to have a dominant frequency display, but this is not available on most equipment. Some displays provide only theta-to-beta ratio information while others can be programmed to give information in any desired format. Session averaging information and statistical report information are especially important, however these reports are often very poorly designed. A quality report will allow the practitioner to take a baseline of any length using any frequency configuration and have instant averaging in a readable format. These reports are not easy to find.

Most equipment is designed for one way of doing neurofeedback. If practitioners want to learn a new approach, they may be forced to buy new equipment in order to operationalize a protocol. One advantage of a simple program based on one approach to neurofeedback is that it is easier to learn, however its narrow approach can be quite limiting. On the other hand, sophisticated programs that offer greater flexibility can be very difficult to learn and easily overwhelm and confuse beginners.

Some manufacturers make a good profit from selling a long series of costly workshops to learn their equipment. We recommend you buy an inexpensive and simple piece of equipment such as those developed by BrainMaster or Pocket Neurobics. You may want to first utilize a basic neurofeedback system, then upgrade to the fancier equipment as you learn more about what you want to do. Later, you can use the simple equipment for backup or as a home trainer. You need to be sure that your equipment complies with federal regulations if you plan to use it for clinical work. This step is extremely important depending on your clinical setting, e.g., a hospital setting in which all medical equipment must meet FDA requirements.

At least two amplifiers are required to do complex bilateral training such as Valdeane Brown's *Period Three* approach. A ratio training format helps if you want to do asymmetry training. Val provides his own complete equipment package, which incorporates high end technology. Multiple tones that sound nice together are important. The ability to program custom tones is an important feature. For example, advanced peak performance training involving synchrony requires a four-channel system.. Until recently, Adam Crane at American Biotech had the only four-channel synchrony program specifically designed for synchrony training. BrainMaster has recently come out with this type of equipment, as well as Thought Technology and Nexus. In addition, lead configuration is important and most equipment can be adapted for bipolar and monopolar montages.

Knowing what type of voltage values are utilized on the equipment, i.e., peak-to-peak[22] or root mean square (RMS)[23] is essential. The voltage readings between machines varies a great deal.. If

---

[22] Peak-to-peak amplitude is the measure of the change between peak and trough. Peak-to-peak amplitudes can be measured by meters with appropriate circuitry, or by viewing the waveform on an oscilloscope. Peak-to-peak is a straightforward measurement to make on an oscilloscope, the peaks of the waveform being easily identified and measured against the graticule. It remains a common way of specifying

you want to compare your voltage readings to others, you need to know each format, so you can adjust for differences. This step is especially important if you are using two different machines or if you want to interpret research.

While no standards exist in the field, more and more machines are using peak-to-peak.

$$RMS = .707 \times peak\ value$$

Other methods are used for calculation of voltage values including average value and peak value.

$$Peak\ to\ Peak\ =\ 2 \times peak\ value.$$

$$2.828 \times RMS = Peak\ to\ Peak.$$

Most machines today have such high input impedance that even if the technique is not great, good readings are still possible. Still, connections should be less than 35 Ohms maximum. Technically, the standard is 5 Ohms. Most of you will have to settle for 10 Ohms. On some equipment there are impedance lights informing you of the connection quality. After some practice, you will usually be able to tell from the readings if the client was prepared properly. When beginning, it is a good idea to get a device to check the resistance of the leads. In this situation, live supervision can help you a great deal and teach you good techniques.

HOOKING IT UP

Reference areas are slightly controversial, but the most common location for reference electrodes is the ear lobes. Some practitioners claim that this location is the only viable placement, but the explanations are not very well documented. Nunez (1995) indicates that there are many equally good locations for ground and reference. For example, many practitioners utilize mastoid references, the boney area behind the ears, with good results. QEEG databases use the ear lobes (linked ears) so it would be best to do so for conformity's sake.

Either one active electrode and one reference electrode with a ground electrode (called monopolar montage) or two active electrodes and a ground electrode (called bipolar montage) is required. The monopolar montage can be utilized with either linked-ears or individual ears. The monopolar montage provides specific local information about a given site. A bipolar montage provides more general regional information.

---

amplitude but sometimes other measures of amplitude are more appropriate (http://en.wikipedia.org/wiki/Amplitude - 01/17/09).

[23] Root mean square (RMS) amplitude is used especially in electrical engineering: the RMS is defined as the square root of the mean over time of the square of the vertical distance of the graph from the rest state. When dealing with alternating current electrical power, it is universal to specify RMS values of a sinusoidal waveform. The peak-to-peak voltage of a sine wave is nearly 3 times the RMS value, but is a rarely used measure in this field (http://en.wikipedia.org/wiki/Amplitude - 01/17/09).

The term linked-ears refers to a condition in which each electrode connected to an ear lobe is linked to the other electrode. The ears are linked together. The rationale behind linking ears is that it should produce the same magnitude readings as a linked-ears database. In addition, the linked-ears electrode arrangement has an added advantage in that it will give more specifically accurate readings at each site; as the clinician moves the so-called "active" electrode over the head, he will get more consistently accurate readings. Since amplitude should theoretically vary with the distance from the reference electrode, having two reference electrodes, one on each side of the head linked together, should compensate for distorted readings due to electrode placement.

The ground is another issue of controversy. Some suggested locations are the ear, the forehead, the nose, the side of the neck, and the back of the neck. Paul Nunez (2006) indicates there is no theoretically superior placement for the ground. Generally, practitioners agree that placement anywhere above the shoulders is good, otherwise cardiac artifact becomes a problem. Using the back of the neck on a bony prominence, the ear lobe, or forehead provides great success.

Note: Most people don't like wires and electrodes on their faces.

Bipolar montages go in and out of fashion frequently. The new correct term, according to Jay Gunkleman (personal communication), is serial montage. Most equipment can be adapted to support this montage. One problem with it is that amplitudes are frequently lower if the electrodes are placed too closely. Some clinicians can be confused by this phenomenon. They may mistakenly compare serial montage baselines with their monopolar baselines and believe that they are getting poor results or that their equipment is malfunctioning. Equipment sensitivity, if not adjustable, may also prove a problem and small readings may be difficult to work with. Training may become almost impossible because amplitude variations are so small. Most modern equipment, however, can compensate for this problem.

In the bipolar, or serial, montage, both reference and active electrodes are placed on the scalp. For instance, one might place one electrode halfway between Fz and Cz and the other halfway between Cz and Pz (Lubar, 1995). This placement was often popular for training ADHD in the 1990s. Interestingly, both of these locations have direct connections with the basal ganglia and directly influence the mesolimbic dopamine system. Margret Ayers often placed one electrode at T3 and another at T4 to increase overall EEG amplitude. She indicated that this placement is dangerous for individuals with family histories of seizure disorder because it increases activity across the corpus callosum. The Othmers presently use this montage extensively with a very complex set of inhibits and enhancements.

THE 10-20 SYSTEM

The standardized system for electrode placement is known as the international 10-20 system (see Chapter Three). Diagram 39: 10-20 International System, page 103, shows the format of this system. It is not necessary to put electrodes only at these placements. The system provides a method of describing where the electrodes are placed when you write notes and/or conduct research. Research indicates that considerable variation occurs between individuals with regard to the association between these locations and underlying brain structures (Homan, Herman, & Purdy, 1987). Consequently, it is not necessary to be too precise with electrode placements unless the brain map indicates a very focal abnormality. If placement is within an area the size of a quarter over a particular site, the 10-20 site will be targeted.

Diagram 39: 10-20 International System

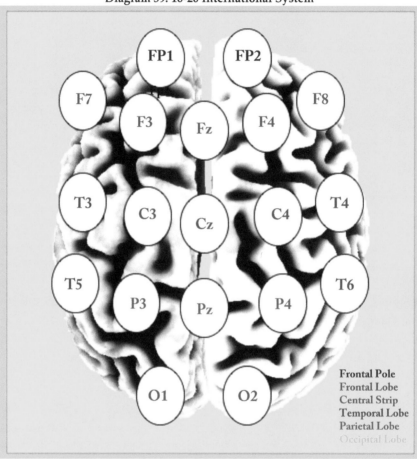

In some cases, you may want to train in different areas besides the 10-20 locations. You should not be afraid to do this with sufficient understanding of the underlying brain anatomy and how it relates to function. Research shows that there can be much variance between the 10-20 system and the underlying structures. So, it is valuable to move the electrode around the area by a factor of 5%-10% (again, about the diameter of a quarter) during each session.

Note: There is also the matter of individual variation in brain structure .

Many people entering the field focus excessively on being precise about electrode placement, but research contradicts this approach. There are, however, some clinicians presently doing coherence training. In this instance, precision may be important because the locations on the brain maps are the actual locations on the client's scalp; however, an error of 3-6 cm is still probably acceptable. The locations have been determined by how the 10-20 system interfaces with that individual's head and are not based on anatomy. The coherence is measured between locations defined by the 10-20 system.

ARTIFACT

Artifact may at first seem a boring subject of unnecessary detail; however, often the session cannot begin until the troublesome artifact is uncovered. When confronted with a client and a time limitation, not being able to determine what is interfering with the readings can be one of the most embarrassing moments in practice. Many novice neurofeedback providers go into a panic when this happens.

Poor connections are usually the source of artifact, which is why there is so much emphasis on good clinical technique. Good technique actually comes from practice more than anything else.

STEPS FOR ELECTRODE PREPARATION AND PLACEMENT

30) Use an alcohol pad and/or abrasive preparation such as Nuprep® to thoroughly wipe the scalp (see Diagram 40, below)

31) Part the hair and hold it down, so that the scalp site is clearly exposed.

32) Maintain control of the hair over the site (this can be difficult) as you try to place the electrode and paste with the other hand.

Note: Make sure there is a pea size dab of paste on the electrode first then ask the client to hold it while you do other things.

Diagram 40: Scalp Preparation, Electrode Preparation, and Placement

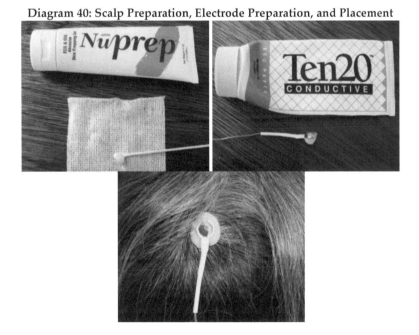

Some novices try to use as little paste as possible to please the client and appease their complaints about how troublesome the glob of paste is in their hair. You need to be firm and remind all involved that this is a clinical procedure and not entertainment. Too little paste is often a major source of trouble. Very short hair will especially prove this point. The bristle of the hair pushs the electrode away from the scalp more so than long hair. Bald heads often require considerable preparation and may need scrubbing with a mild abrasive (i.e., Nuprep) at the site. Special abrasive pads/skin wipes (—see Appendix A, page 173) can also be used for this procedure.

Poor connections can result in too much amplitude in some frequency domains and too little in others. For example:

- A poor ground connection can result in very high measures and wild swings in EEG amplitudes.
- Poor reference electrode connections usually look like there is too little amplitude, as does poor active electrode connections. There also often appears to be a very elevated beta with a poor active electrode.
- Eye blinks frequently cause large excursions of the EEG, especially in the low frequency domain. Some individuals will register eye blinks as far back on their scalp as Cz. Some individuals move their eyes around a lot as well. This movement looks like smaller hills in the EEG.
- Too much heat coming off the scalp causes excursions that look like hills in the raw EEG.
- Beware of gum chewers and those who grit their teeth when they focus intently, as this will increase general amplitude.

With some children, it is necessary to put an EMG electrode on their jaw muscles to make sure they are not producing what looks like wonderful results by clenching the jaw. Some people generate deviations in EEG when they swallow; this motion also shows up especially well in low frequencies. Diagram 41, page 104, shows EEG artifact due to physical movement. To become acquainted with all of them, you should hook the equipment up to yourself. It is well worth the time and effort.

In addition, variation due to head structure and scalp tension exists. Too much scalp tension generates elevated beta frequency that can be very deceptive. Often, when people are training, they will unknowingly tense up their scalp muscles and appear to produce incredible amplitudes of beta. Sometimes the effect is so subtle that it is difficult to tell if beta increases are artifact or scalp tension. Putting an EMG electrode on the scalp (some equipment has built-in scalp tension sensors that automatically invalidate any data that is tainted) can often help identify the difference (if there is a difference). By watching the parallel activity in the beta range and the EMG range, practitioners can roughly assess how much of the signal is EMG. A helpful approach is to work on relaxing the scalp and see how low clients can get their EMG. Over several trials, the clinician can get a sense of what component of the beta is scalp tension and coach clients to stay relaxed during training.

Diagram 41: EEG Artifact Due to Physical Movement

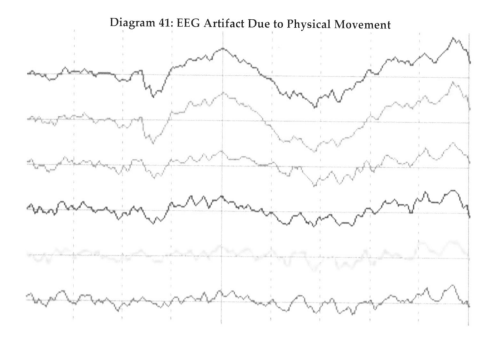

THE SUDDEN RISE AND FALL OF WAVES IS INDICATIVE OF MOVEMENT

It is interesting to note that some clinicians aren't convinced that people can learn to appreciably increase beta amplitudes and suspect that perhaps practitioners are just conditioning scalp muscles. Both Barry Sterman and Marvin Sams (personal communication) are convinced that beta is very unreliable and not to be trusted. When training at New Mind, we focus on observing theta reduction even though we may be telling the client to increase beta. We note that during efforts to increase beta, they usually decrease theta first. In fact, Margaret Ayers and Barry Sterman (personal communication) focus more on theta reduction techniques rather than beta enhancement. Many clients can learn to decrease their EEG just as easily, or more easily, than they can learn to increase it. In many cases, this action is preferable. Overall, it is easier to work with slow waves, even though much of the general artifact shows up in these ranges. It is important to watch the client and check to see if the artifact is an eye blink or body movement, being careful because most clients get very uncomfortable when observed too intently.

Feedback usually occurs within 60-100 ms, based on equipment response times. Considerable training occurs between eye blinks and other periodic artifacts. Our clinical experience shows that good results still ensue.

Clinicians using Z-score training may have more varied results. Just how much artifact interferes with Z-score training is not yet clear. In the meantime, it is best to avoid frontal lead artifact as much as possible. One of the best ways to do this is to keep impedances low through good electrode contact.

Some clients register a heartbeat in their EEG. This can be difficult to eliminate, but moving the ground to a location higher up the neck or onto the forehead or nose can reduce it considerably. Increasing the time constant or sample rate (also called averaging or damping) of the equipment can help filter out the rhythmic changes in the EEG enough for training purposes. Some individuals, such as those with chronic headache, have such high EMG that on many occasions their EEG is impossible to record or train. They often average upper body EMGs in the range of 25 μV or higher.

For example, one client completely scrambled our signal almost every session. We frequently concluded that our equipment was faulty because all of our connections were perfect. We checked and rechecked everything and were about to give up training her when we found out that the right side of her face frequently went numb. Like so many other clients, she never told us this important fact—it wasn't on the intake form. One day, she came in complaining of this condition. We put the EMG electrode on that side of her face. The EMG showed that all her muscles were in spasm, so we trained her to gain control of those muscles and relax them. Once that was done, we were able to get a good EEG signal.

Since then, we have found that some clients come in with so much EMG that their EEG cannot be trained until relaxation training is successful. Once they get more control over their EMG, this situation ceases to be a problem. This is another reason why we like to begin clients with a few sessions of alpha training. They learn to relax in the office chair and produce fewer artifacts. Thus, in some cases, relaxation training may be indicated before a patient is started in neurofeedback.

Sometimes individuals may come in with contact lens problems and/or allergy problems that cause them to blink and swallow a lot. and you will be forced to move your electrode to more posterior areas of the scalp or have the client train with eyes closed. There is some indication that training with eyes open and eyes closed affects the brain differently; however, there isn't enough research to verify this. It is worthwhile to look for individual differences in this area in order to compensate, if necessary. We generally train adolescents with eyes open. With adults, we may ask a preference, and when possible, accommodate them.

DON'T PANIC

Novice neurofeedback trainers often panic as the hour goes by and they cannot isolate the problem with their equipment. They often look less than competent in the new client's eyes. However, the more aroused they become, the poorer problem solvers they become, and they overlook important details. Instead, they need to go through the connections methodically starting with the most common problems and then considering the more rare ones. It is helpful to put the client on audio visual entrainment (AVE) when these problems occur. Less time is wasted, and it doesn't interfere with the problem-solving efforts. Under these conditions, it is even possible to make a phone call to the manufacturer and ask questions without losing client confidence. In addition, obtaining one-on-one troubleshooting training and drilling is a good idea.

TAKING BASELINES

Baselines are controversial. Some clinicians only take baselines at the outset of treatment and after long intervals of training. Others say that they are almost useless; still others demand a QEEG every ten sessions. The Othmers have a huge database on baselines before and after training and have noticed very little change in many individual baselines despite dramatic changes in behavior. So what is actually changing, if this is the case?

The argument has often been made that mostly responsivity, or plasticity, is changing under cognitive load. That is to say, the way the EEG looks when the brain is performing a task is changing. Therefore, a better measure of change is training performance. To deal with this controversy, Lubar (1995) averages baseline and training averages together. The results appear useful, but the reasoning may not hold up under close scrutiny.

Diagram 42: One-Month Cycle: Alpha (7-10) Baselines in Microvolts, below shows how the baseline varied in one client. In her case, the baseline EEG shifted as much as 8 microvolts from session to session within the same week. The diagram shows only the variation in the alpha amplitudes, but other frequency component bands shifted similarly. It is interesting to note that the client's frontal alpha was consistently high on Tuesday and low on Thursday. Overall, the baseline amplitude decreased over the month, possibly due to the training. As mentioned before, this is not always the case, but in this instance baseline was a good measure of symptom improvement and correlated with it. The chart below shows the baseline blood pressure drop as the baseline alpha dropped.

Diagram 42: One-Month Cycle: Alpha (7-10) Baselines in Microvolts

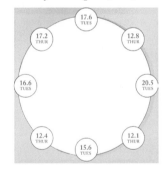

Hz	T	Th	T	Th	T	Th	T	Th
	4/22	4/24	4/29	5/8	5/13	5/15	5/20	5/22
4-6	7.1	6.1	7.2	6.5	9.6	6.3	6.9	6.9
7-10	17.6	12.8	20.5	12.1	15.6	12.4	16.6	17.2
15-30	14.9	14.0	14.7	14.1	19.0	13.6	15.3	14.9
BP	----	----	190/117	---	---	163/107	---	158/106

The client's depression shifted into the normal range as well. If a baseline had not been taken at each session and instead the alpha threshold had been set consistently at 15 microvolts, one would have the impression that she was doing a better job of training her alpha down on Thursdays than on Tuesdays. This could have led to making the training too difficult on Tuesdays and she would have not trained as well (due to ratio strain).

In the past, many clinicians have taken a baseline at just Cz alone. Michael Tansey (Lubar Workshop) obtains tremendous results doing SMR training at Cz alone. The Othmers tend to take their baselines at C3, Cz, and C4. This process is arguably a limited picture of the brain's EEG activity and perhaps explains why QEEG specialists see changes. They may be seeing more subtle shifts due to the resolution of their database. In spite of rumors to the contrary, those of us using QEEG do see changes and usually in the expected direction. These changes are not as dramatic as was once expected early in the development of the field, but research has shown that the brain doesn't get rid of old networks, it builds new networks. The changes are going to be more subtle in many cases rather than dramatically returning to some theoretical norm.

In our experience, we have often seen greater changes in coherence than in spectral distribution and amplitude. Either way, it is the client's subjective perspective that counts most in the end. If the client feels better and symptoms are diminishing, then the brain is changing. When doing research, it is clearly best to use QEEGs; however, many clinicians do fine with monopolar analysis.

MONOPOLAR ANALYSIS: THE MINI Q

Monopolar exploration can be used almost as effectively as QEEG. If the norm for Cz is known, you can almost predict what the brain map is going to show generally, due to volume conduction, by taking five or six readings at different basic sites. Careful monopolar exploration around other areas of the scalp can further confirm initial observations of possible emerging patterns. This approach, however, works best with the right kind of EEG equipment, a good working knowledge of neurophysiology, and considerable prior experience or training in what to look for.

Diagram 44: EEG Distributions, page 112 shows the baseline profile for young, healthy adults drawn from a research article. As mentioned in the section on instrumentation, EEG equipment varies a great deal among models and manufacturers regarding sensitivity and method of calculation of voltage amplitude. Individuals also have stronger EEGs in their youth and usually produce less power as they age. Another problem is skull thickness, which can alter amplitude readings considerably, i.e., the thicker the skull, the lower the amplitude.

Because of this tremendous variation, the neurology community was initially skeptical of the value of QEEG, and still is. E. Roy John (1988), however, has demonstrated a strong consistency in EEGs across cultures and age groups for normal individuals and has found a method to calculate a useful database. Hershel Toomim (personal communication) has long been a champion of looking at beta-to-theta ratios to offset this problem in another way. By calculating the ratios among all standard frequency ranges (component bands) in normative individuals, those ratios can be used as an indicator of EEG deviance by comparing them with ratios of other individuals.

Diagram 43: Estimated Standard Deviations of Magnitude at Cz (Eyes-Closed)

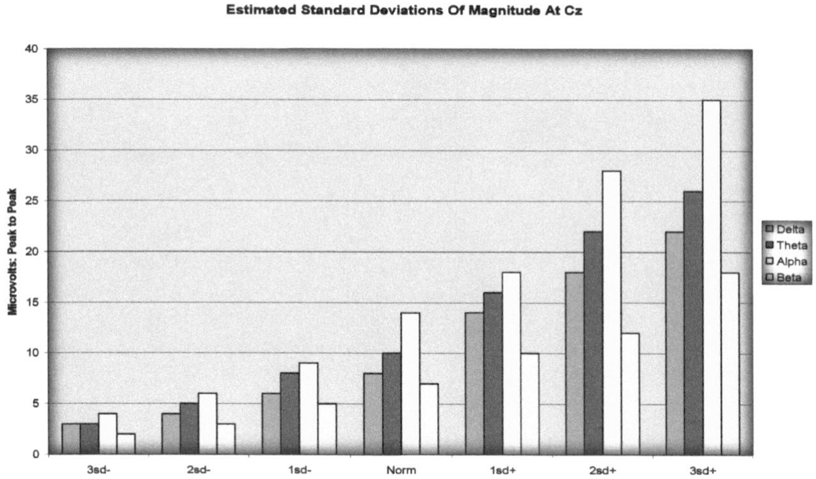

Estimated Standard Deviations Of Magnitude At Cz

REVIEW

It is often useful to look at the brain in terms of front vs. back and left vs. right. The brain should be running faster in the front and slower in the back. It should also be running faster on the left than on the right. At Cz, research indicates that with eyes closed, alpha should be highest with theta about 2/3 of alpha and beta ½ to 1/3 of alpha. Brain maps indicate that the ratio should shift slightly as you move forward toward FPz with beta becoming progressively higher and alpha and theta becoming progressively lower. The ratio should also shift backwards with beta and theta diminishing and alpha increasing. By taking a baseline at Fz, and perhaps FPz, you can watch for a trend. If theta is increasing, then ADHD may be present. If alpha is increasing, then depression may be present. If beta increases dramatically, then anxiety is possible.

By taking a baseline at Pz, you can look for similar trends. If theta increases dramatically, then repressed trauma is possible. If beta increases, intense emotionality related to anxiety is possible. When moving toward the occipital cortex, alpha should increase.

Taking readings at C3 and C4 allows you to compare differences in hemispheric symmetry. Anxiety, depression, and ADHD have definite bilateral signatures. Anxiety and especially mania,tend to push beta to the right. According to Davidson (1995), depression usually shows as alpha higher on the left side than the right. Bob Gurnee (personal communication) finds that high alpha in the right frontal area is associated with a subtype of ADHD. Other research relates high frontal theta or alpha to OCD in some cases (see Chapter Three).

Eyes-open frontal theta or alpha can also indicate ADHD or depression. If you ask a client to perform backward serial 7s, that is, count backward from 100 by 7s, and the client's alpha or theta increases, then you are likely dealing with ADHD. Clients can read or do a computerized performance test and show the same phenomenon. Many individuals with depression have very low eyes-open alpha, but very high eyes-closed alpha (three-to-one ratio)—even at Cz. When brain maps are evaluated, alpha is almost always found in the 7-8 Hz range. Alpha in the low 9 Hz range is more often found in cases of damage to the frontal area due to toxic exposure or excess use of amphetamines or cocaine derivatives. It frequently looks like ADHD on the testing and this frequency has been found dominant in one case with drug-related psychosis. We have seen elevated SMR in over a dozen cases of mycotoxin exposure[24] (How many cases?) along with a great deal of global slowing with very low amplitudes in the beta range. We have seen a similar pattern in some seizure disorders. Interestingly, coherence was not relivantly abnormal in these cases.

If the equipment allows you to look at frequency in some form of spectral display, you will find that anxiety varies in appearance between excess 16 to 20 Hz to excess 23 to 30 Hz. The lower 16-20 Hz range is referred to as the "beta ridge" by the Lubars (personal communication). It often shows up in individuals who are very controlling and argumentative. In addition, they often have a lot of physical symptoms, especially severe sleep problems. The 23-30 Hz range tends to show up more as a hyper-vigilant type of anxiety.

Focal areas of high theta or delta are often related to local tissue damage.

According to Thatcher (personal communication, 1997, 1998), the delta is related to white matter damage and the theta to grey matter damage. If this baseline is found, we recommend not proceeding without a QEEG.

These baselines provide clear indicators of where to train. Although not as accurate as a QEEG, they closely predict what the maps will show. The most difficult frequency to assess in this manner is beta. Small changes in beta can be meaningful, but hard to recognize. The beta-to-theta ratio is often a good indicator of the stregnth of the beta level.

The baselines can be checked regularly as clients are treated without sacrificing a great deal of time and expense. Dramatic changes can be seem in bilateral baselines and performance averages. Large global changes, on the other hand, tend to occur very slowly over time. Sometimes they are not visible for a year or so.

---

[24] Aflatoxins are naturally occurring mycotoxins that are produced by many species of Aspergillus, a fungus. Aflatoxins are toxic and among the most carcinogenic substances known (http://en.wikipedia.org/wiki/Aflatoxin - 01/18/08).

Diagram 44: EEG Distributions

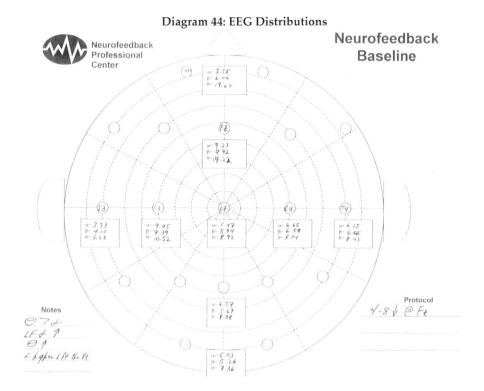

Diagram 44: EEG Distributions (above) is a sample single-electrode eyes-closed brain map. When starting with Cz, it is apparent that alpha is lower than beta or theta, which is abnormal for the eyes-closed condition. In terms of anterior to posterior amplitude (i.e., in front of and behind the sensorimotor strip, theta clearly decreases in the posterior direction and increases as you move frontally from 8.92 to 17.64 by the time you reach Fpz. This individual is clearly ADHD with too much frontal theta. Beta at Fz is 4.92 while it is 5.67 at Pz, which is also abnormal.

Research finds correlations between intense emotions and posterior beta. Many clinicians find posterior beta present in anxiety as well. In this case, you will see that beta is higher in the right temporal area than in the left, which suggests anxiety.

Note: Alpha also increases somewhat frontally, suggesting the presence of depression.

If you check the asymmetry between left and right hemispheres, you will see that the alpha is 6.65 on the right and 9.05 on the left. Clearly, alpha is highest on the left, which is consistent with depression. Theta is much higher on the left as well. The left hemisphere is under-activated.

In this example, we decided to start with theta suppression at Fz. If such a client does not respond well to this protocol, we might try dealing with the depression first by up-training alpha in the right hemisphere or beta in the left hemisphere. Every client varies in his or her response to a protocol, which is why neurofeedback is not a cut-and-dried process.

BASIC PREPARATION

When planning to conduct a QEEG on patients, there are a few basic instructions to follow. QEEGs are best conducted in the morning vs. afternoon, i.e., between the hours of 9:00 a.m. and 1:00 p.m. Many experts insist on avoiding caffeine, but many people are habituated to caffeine, with associated neurophysiological changes. Avoiding it may actually distort their "usual" record. With no caffeine, more drowsiness and slowing may be present in the record, whereas with the caffeine, they may demonstrate a more normal record because of their habituation. On the other hand, too much caffeine may also distort the record with excessive fast-wave activity. In this case, moderation is likely to give the most accurate record.

If the patient is taking stimulant medication (i.e., ADHD medication), it is preferable to do the QEEG after the patient has not taken the medication for 48 hours. The patient MUST check with his/her prescribing physician to determine if it is possible to stop taking the stimulants 48 hours prior to the QEEG. If a break of 48 hours is not advisable, a break of 24 hours is the next preferred length, and a break of 12-24 hours is the next preferred length after that. Do not make changes in any other medication (unless authorized by the patient's physician). Follow these steps:

33) If the patient is sick, instruct him or her to call to reschedule, even if he or she only has a cold.

34) The patient should not drink coffee, tea, Red Bull, caffeinated soft drinks, or any other substance with caffeine for at least 15 hours prior to the QEEG.

Note: If the patient drinks coffee or caffeinated beverages in the morning, then stopping caffeine may affect the outcome of the QEEG. Over time, individuals may habituate to a mild stimulus such as regular coffee and develop a physiological adaptation. For instance, not drinking the usual amount of coffee may result in headaches and fogginess that generate an abnormal EEG pattern with increased alpha slowing and/or increased scalp EMG. This may accentuate the EEG abnormalities more than the coffee. More research needs to be done in this area to clarify these kinds of confounds.

35) Patients should avoid taking any over-the-counter medication or supplements for three to four days prior to the QEEG. This includes vitamins.

36) The patient should be instructed to wash his or her hair the night before the QEEG by doing the following:

   a)   Wash hair 3 times with a pH neutral cleansing/clarifying shampoo, such as Neutrogena non-residue shampoo.
   b)   Do not use crème rinse or any other hair product prior to the QEEG appointment.
   c)   Do not wash hair again in the morning of the appointment.
   d)   Make sure hair is completely dry before coming for the QEEG.

37) The patient should be instructed to get a good night's sleep before the QEEG (let the practitioner know if there are any sleep problems or disturbances); six or more hours of sleep are preferred.

The day of the QEEG, the patient should:

38) Eat a high-protein breakfast.

39) Drink plenty of water.

40) Use the restroom just prior to the start of the QEEG.

When conducting a QEEG, you should always begin with eyes-closed measures.

TESTING

Testing is not always necessary, since clients frequently arrive with a diagnosis. However, it can be very helpful for a variety of reasons. Clients often arrive with a diagnosis that may or may not be accurate. Often they self-diagnose and present their diagnosis as if it were professionally derived. On the other hand, diagnostic categories do not always correlate with EEG patterns. One protocol does not always work best with a specific disorder. Because of these problems, it is not a good idea to rely too much on diagnostic categories for treatment plans.

For neurofeedback, an EEG analysis is more important. Since symptoms are usually being treated, it is more important to have a list of specific symptoms and problem behaviors. The symptom and behavioral changes guide the practitioner. Using a symptom tracking system is helpful to track changes over time.

Monitoring session progress helps show changes to the client, so clients can see their progress. Often the changes are very subtle for the first ten sessions. Many clients may not even be aware of the changes taking place until 20 or 30 sessions. Even then, they may not recognize that changes have been happening until they have changed a great deal. In fact, others around them often notice the changes first. For this reason, it is important to involve those who are close to the the client to observe the changes and make comments.

The tests we use are the TOVA (or IVA), the Beck Depression Inventory, the Interactive Self Inventory (ISI) or Personality Assessment Inventory (PAI), and Microcog. Recently, we have developed a subjective questionnaire that generates a predictive brain map. It can be accessed on our website at www.newmindmaps.com. This questionnaire can help clinicians determine which locations should be reviewed with the greatest scrutiny on the actual brain map with respect to symptomology.

These tests are not especially long or expensive. They cover basic areas of change such as mood, cognitive functioning, and personality. Recently at New Mind, we added the Integ Neuro comprehensive neurological screening system (www.brainresource.com). We use this test especially for individuals with TBI. It integrates dozens of neurological tests into a single one-hour test that is performed on an IBM kiosk screen and is mostly nonverbal. This test is a major step forward, since it can supply much of the same information quickly and easily that would otherwise be obtained over several days of one-on-one testing by a specialist.

The clinician determines the frequency and administration of all these tests. To demonstrate change, some individuals require more objective measures than others, depending on how much self-awareness they have in the beginning. Others may require the tests for review by other professionals, such as medical doctors or lawyers. We have especially relied on the TOVA and Beck Depression Inventory in the past. The Interactive Self Inventory, which we developed, provides us with much of this information in one package, including information on personal interaction style that can confound training outside of the office environment.

The Othmers should also be commended for developing a short TOVA-like test, the Quick Test. This test can be conducted at the end of each session for session-to-session evaluation. With these new emerging tests designed especially for the neurofeedback practitioner, the clinician should find his or her job much easier in today's clinical environment.

Diagram 45: T.O.V.A. below contains an example of the targets used in the TOVA. They flash on the computer screen in a relatively random pattern. Clients must click on a button, which they hold in one hand, when the target appears and avoid clicking when the non-target appears. The test is nonverbal in nature and lasts 22 minutes.

The test records the following:

- missed targets (omissions)
- clicked non-targets (comissions)
- consistency and response time

This test provides a very good measure of attention and is sensitive to how it is impacted by ADD, depression, and anxiety. Since it is normed, relatively quick, and inexpensive, it is a good objective measure of progress in neurofeedback training. The IVA is a similar test that integrates auditory testing with the visual test and is also available to neurofeedback clinicians.

Diagram 45: T.O.V.A.

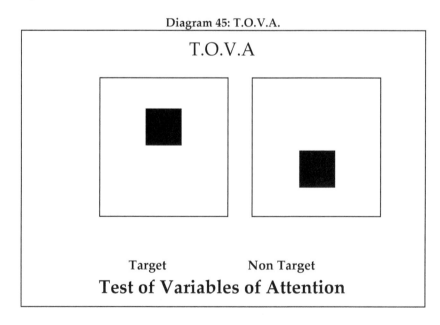

Using Tests Together

One client came to us with problems of memory, concentration, and complaints that she might be less than intelligent. This client had trouble getting motivated. Her EEG showed very high amplitude eyes-closed low frequency alpha. We often find that this situation is an indicator of depression or ADD. In order to distinguish between the two disorders, we gave her the above combination of tests.

Before testing, we made sure there was no history of head injury. Her TOVA showed a mild attentional difficulty, but not ADHD. The Microcog indicated normal intelligence, but poor short-term memory function. The Beck Depression Inventory confirmed problems with anxiety and some mild depression. We showed her the tests and explained that the short-term memory deficit was likely a result of chronic anxiety. The prolonged over-arousal of her sympathetic nervous system had generated so much cortisol that she had experienced degradation in her hippocampal tissue. We then began training her for the depression that likely developed as a result of chronic anxiety. (Beta training at C3 often works well, and sometimes we use asymmetry alpha training as well.)

We have had other clients who were only interested in a reduction of symptoms and didn't see the value of the tests. To deal with this kind of client, we use a subjective symptom checklist that the client fills out at the beginning of each session.. Through self-reporting, clients easily see progressive changes. This process sensitizes them to their own changes and provides us with a way to go back and show them what they themselves have observed in the course of their own training. A sample of this checklist can be found in Appendix D: Forms on page 175.

Clinical Etiquette

Most clinicians are familiar with the rules of clinical etiquette; however, issues arise unique to neurofeedback that should be discussed.

Creating the Environment

Managing the environment so that it is a relaxed and predictable atmosphere is important. When clients are alpha training or theta training, it is important to keep the room quiet and avoid all distractions. Eliminating ringing phones or other intrusions is critical. Making sure the client's chair is comfortable and adequate and maintaining a comfortable room temperature are important. Having a fan present can help clients avoid getting overheated. For example, when clients get too hot, the electrode paste tends to melt, distorting signals as electrodes come loose and fall off. A blanket for individuals with poor peripheral vascularity may also be helpful. However, during beta or SMR uptraining, distractions are actually helpful challenges to client training.

Developing Routines

Practitioners should develop a set routine to avoid upsetting sensitive clients. Explaining each step of the routine before it is performed helps clients until they are familiar with the protocol.

Explaining Neurofeedback

Because of the nature of neurofeedback training, many practitioners find clients complaining that they don't understand what they are doing, or asking, "How am I doing this?" Clients may often say, "I still don't get how this works." Although clients would never question a pill or the mechanics of anesthetics, the neurofeedback environment is so novel and alien to their way of thinking that it is difficult for them to accept what is going on until they experience a dramatic change.

It is a good idea to develop a series of well-rehearsed short answers that can become more complex as the knowledge of the client grows. Clients frequently want something to read regarding neurofeedback and its efficacy. At New Mind, we often give them scientific research, which they happily accept even though most of them do not have the training to interpret the research. Providing client-friendly brochures may be more helpful. The World Wide Web can also be a good tool because clients can access detailed explanations from your own site and/or other sites at any time.

Recognizing Changes

To help clients recognize changes, you should discuss expected changes before training begins. Clients are very likely to attribute changes to other factors at first. Changes in response to stressors and sleep patterns are among the first that they notice. Asking about symptoms at each session will help keep track of changes, so you can support client observations and assist them in arriving at their own conclusions based on their own observations. It often takes an extended period before they realize that the changes are permanent and likely due to the neurofeedback.

Note: Problems may arise if expected changes are emphasized too much, because many clients will believe that change is due to the placebo effect.

Audio Visual Entrainment or AVE is a tremendous help for managing clients. When they come in overtired and falling asleep during training, a ten-minute AVE nap can refresh them and get them working effectively at training again. When they look for something dramatic during the first few sessions, AVE provides them with the stimulation they seek. They are often more willing to accept the efficacy of AVE at the outset because it is so dramatic. Interestingly, in our experience, clients ask fewer questions regarding it.

Results from AVE are usually short-lived but dramatic, and clients are excited about the training. This helps them focus on the NFB more. Eventually they realize on their own that the effects of the NFB are more profound and longer lasting. Clients then shift their enthusiasm over to NFB with fewer questions and complaints.

Problem Clients

Occasionally clients are confrontational and suspicious and their questions reflect this. This situation often happens with individuals with personality disorders or with severely depressed clients who harbor considerable anger. Until clients experience dramatic changes in their conditions, this needs to be delicately managed, which requires more patience on the part of the clinician than with other clients. Patient and consistent responses with firm reassurances are often necessary and most effective.

For example, should you be challenged by a client at every session in a way that undermines your confidence, it is possible that the client has borderline personality disorder. These individuals require a practitioner with considerable clinical skill. It is best to refer them to someone who his this expertise Importanlly, these clients may be prone to legal action. Personality tests at the outset can be a great help in identifying this type of client.

Note: Do not engage in argument with clients. Refer to more experienced clinicians if necessary.

Drug Effects on EEG

A fair amount of literature is available on this topic. It is important to know this information to better assess the baseline analysis of clients. Table 9: Drug Effects on EEG, page 119, lists the drugs most frequently encountered that have a significant effect on EEG.

Recently, it has come to our attention that benzodiazepines can confound training with NFB— especially alpha-theta training. Many people using these drugs are either addicted to them or experiencing a long withdrawal and recovery period. Some psychiatrists even refuse to work with them. Typically, training someone who is on SSRIs or methylphenidate derivatives does not retard training results, but some newer drugs appear to have this capacity.

Family	Drugs	Purpose	EEG Impact
Neuroleptics	Haldol, Prolixin, Thorazine, Mellaril	Sedative	Increase delta, theta and beta above 20 Hz and decrease alpha and beta below 20 Hz.
Neuroleptics	Seroquel, Risperdal, Geodone	Non-sedative and antipsychotic medications	Decrease alpha and increase beta in general.
Anxiolytics	Valium, Halcion, Librium, Dalmane	Anxiety relief	Decrease alpha and increase beta, especially 13-20 Hz beta
Benzodiazepines	Valium, Xanax, and Ativan	Anxiety, panic relief	Decrease alpha and increase 20-30 Hz beta
SSRIs	Prozac, Paxil, and Zoloft	a class of antidepressants used in the treatment of depression, anxiety disorders, and some personality disorders.	Decrease in frontal alpha and a mild increase in 18-25 Hz beta.
MAO Inhibitors	Marplan, Parnate, Eldepryl	Antidepressant	Tendency to increase 20-30 Hz beta while decreasing all other frequencies
Tricyclic antidepressants	Imipramine and Amitriptyline	Useful in depressed patients with insomnia, restlessness, and nervousness	Increase delta and theta while decreasing alpha; increase beta 25 Hz and up band
Antipsychotics	Lithium	Used for the treatment of manic/depressive (bipolar) and depressive disorders	Increases theta, mildly decreases alpha and increases beta
Amphetamines	Adderall, Vyvanse, and Dexedrine.	a group of drugs that act by increasing levels of norepinephrine, serotonin, and dopamine in the brain	Decrease slow-wave activity and increase beta in the 12-26 Hz range
Marijuana		Recreational	Increases frontal low frequency alpha; affects EEG for three days
Opiates	Opium, hydromorphone, oxymorphone, heroin, morphine, oxycodone, Talwin, codeine, methadone, meperdine, hydrocodone, Vicodin	Pain relief	Generate high amplitude slow alpha in the 8 Hz range
Barbiturates	Brevital, thiamylal (Surital), thiopental (Pentothal), amobarbital, Amytal, pentobarbital, Nembutal, secobarbital, Seconal, Tuinal, Phenobarbital, Luminal, mephobarbital, Mebaral	Produce a wide spectrum of central nervous system depression, from mild sedation to coma, and have been used as sedatives, hypnotics, anesthetics, and anticonvulsants	Increase beta at 25-35 Hz amplitude
Caffeine		Increases alertness	Increases beta and decreases slower waves

REVIEW QUESTIONS

41) What is Ohm's law?

42) What is impedance?

43) What are $E = I \times R$; $V = R \times I$; $I = V/R$; and $R = V/I$?

44) What effect do barbiturates have on the brain?

45) What is common mode rejection?

46) What are the differences between a low-pass filter and a high-pass filter?

47) What is a fast Fourier transform?

48) What effects are seen from opiates?

49) What is a standard deviation from Cz?

LEARNING THEORY AND EEG TRAINING

Neurofeedback training is a form of operant conditioning and to some degree classical conditioning as well. It is important to know the basics regarding these two subjects and a basic psychology text can refresh your memory. It is crucial to maintain a specific range of reinforcement rate for optimal training and results. In addition, the type and pitch of sound is important. Another factor to consider is proportional vs. dichotomous types of reinforcement.

Most instructions suggest setting thresholds so that enhancement reinforcement rates are at 75% and inhibition rates at 25%. However, we use several different brands of EEG equipment and have not found these settings to be appropriate for any of them or for our clients either. In fact, our databases confirm our observations. Setting thresholds so that reinforcement rates are in the range of 80% to 90% often produces much better performance. Inhibition amplitudes are better if reinforcement is around 10% to 20% in the positive direction or an inhibition reward of 80% to 90%. In other words, most equipment will read 20% on the inhibitory filter. This means the client will be reinforced for being below threshold 80% of the time.

If practitioners deviate very far from these settings, ratio strain occurs. This means that the reinforcement rate is too low to be rewarding to clients, and they don't make as good an effort. So it isn't worth the time. This situation has very little to do with conscious motivation of the client. Even the most motivated client does not do as well when ratio strain occurs, proving once again the validity of behavioristic research.

Note: Reinforcement rates have to be adjusted differently for the same person on different pieces of equipment. For instance, individuals who perform best at 75% on Thought Technology® equipment perform best at 60% on the BrainMaster® equipment.

TYPES OF REINFORCEMENT

Dichotomous reinforcement occurs when clients receive feedback in the form of a sound, image, or both, when they exceed a given threshold. In some cases, they may receive reinforcement only when they stay below a given threshold. Clients either meet the criteria or they don't. There is also equipment on the market that provides constant reinforcement of images and sound. It is constant and ongoing because it informs clients of their performance through pitch variance or image changes. This method is called proportional feedback. Joe Kamiya's (personal communication) research on reinforcement and training indicates that constant proportional reinforcement is superior to dichotomous.

With proportional reinforcement, it is usually better not to set a threshold at all—just tell the client to do the best he or she can. We have also found that the range of pitch of the tone being used for reinforcement is crucial. Lower pitched tones reduce performance. Humans respond better to higher pitched tones when trying to increase their amplitudes. In addition, when training with eyes open, providing training graphs with wave forms displayed near the top of the graph increases reinforcement. With dichotomous reinforcement, such factors don't play a crucial role; however, a pleasing tone increases reinforcement more than a harsh tone.

OPTIMAL TRAINING

This brings us to optimal reinforcement in particular. Travis et al. (1974) also found in their research that 10-minute intervals were optimal for training alpha and that one could run three 10-minute intervals in one sitting; proportional or non-dichotomous training was most effective. We have found it true as well and also include beta in that category. On the other hand, optimal training times for theta appear to be 20 to 30 minutes. It is routine for us to do most of our training in the form of 3- to 7-minute trials (7 minutes is the average attention span of an adult). Pushing clients beyond these considerations appears counterproductive when we evaluate the performance data post session. It is important to provide clients with a rest between trials. Data indicates they usually become tired and begin performing more poorly after the third trial.

Many neurotherapists find that there is no limit to frequency of training. Research published by Bill Scott et al. (2005) showed empirically that training individuals twice a day every day for 14 days could normalize a TOVA. This method is great for a client with unlimited funds flying in from out of town who wants to get the job done right away. However, realistically, most individuals respond well to a twice-a-week schedule.

Physiological changes take place between sessions and neural growth takes time and cannot be pushed beyond a reasonable limit. However, individuals need time to adjust their lives to the changes taking place in their brains. Dysfunctional networks take years to grow and it will probably take a year or two to undo the damage even if training takes only several weeks or 3 months. The match between these two factors has not been adequately researched. However, we find that people continue to experience profound changes even a year after training, which supports theories regarding *initial conditions* from a chaotic systems perspective.

In spite of all our innovation and efforts to try out everybody's protocols, we still find that most people require at least 30-40 sessions (even with Z-score training) to solidify their gains, even if they experience dramatic gains in the first 15 sessions. Once initial gains are made in the first 10 to 20 sessions, frequency of visits can be reduced. Our records indicate that progress is slowed considerably if clients only come once a week at the outset.

Another valuable tool is audio-visual entrainment (AVE). Chapter Nine explains how to use AVE. If used in conjunction with NFB, AVE enhances performance dramatically. By using it in between NFB trials, practitioners can provide clients time to rest while their brains are passively trained to do the task. An analogy often used is that AVE is to EEG as training wheels are to a bike when learning to ride. After AVE, clients begin the next trial refreshed and usually perform much better. Sometimes the difference is dramatic. They also find the training sessions more enjoyable and look forward to them more. On occasion, when they are sleep deprived, AVE provides them with the opportunity to catnap while also getting entrained. This method also enhances performance on the next trial and provides a good training session that otherwise might have been wasted trying to keep clients awake.

PROTOCOL DETERMINATION

NFB Complexity

Unfortunately, NFB deals with a complex structure and system. Protocol selection is one of the greatest mysteries of NFB and also one of the most intimidating areas for those practitioners just starting out. People entering the field want clear guidelines to assure they are doing the right thing. Many practitioners are frustrated and impatient with the complexity and vagueness of this topic. Trying to generate subtle shifts in that system is a daunting task. However, there is the "Church of the 14 Hz" as Julian Issacs has called it (personal communication).

The NFB pioneer Michael Tansey (Lubar Workshop) found that he could treat almost any disorder effectively if he up-trained a person at 14 Hz at Cz long enough. Although this is not always true, in many cases it is an effective approach. On the other hand, it could cause serious problems if the individual had too much 14 Hz to begin with. Nevertheless, the idea of a few simple protocols that can be used systematically is very appealing to clinicians. This is one reason why the Othmers' initial approach to NFB is so popular. It is very simple and systematic, even if they have not always been sure of why it worked or why practitioners should ignore other alternatives, such as QEEG or Val Brown's approach. Sue Othmer has completely changed her method and protocols over the years and now "different" is good!

Of course there are a dozen other high-profile figures in the field claiming that their ways are the best ways and all the methods work pretty well. Still, many newcomers to the field shake their heads and say "How can this be? It must be placebo." For them, it is necessary to go back and read the research, especially Sterman's research on training cats to produce SMR, where he increases their resistance to the toxic effects of hydrazine fuel. In our opinion, the research proves that success in NFB is not attributable to placebo and shows there are over 2500 therapeutic methods in the field of psychology.

Many trainers prefer to begin at the motor strip. Margaret Ayers (personal communication) believed that it is the best place to start. She worked outward from that point, depending on the problem. The Othmers (personal communication in several workshops) state that the largest and oldest pyramidal cells are in the motor strip area, so it is easiest to influence thalamic oscillators from this area. They even begin with their newer protocols largely from this same starting point. Lubar (personal communication) did a lot of his training with a bipolar montage that extends from Fz back to Pz. Some of his research suggests that training in one area can influence quite a wide region of the brain. Valdeane Brown's (personal communication in several workshops) protocols are usually done along the motor strip as well, C3 and C4, although he has begun to expand this repertoire. Another reason for the popularity of this area is that it is relatively artifact free. It is very difficult to train in front of the motor strip with eyes open because this region is often contaminated by eye-blink artifact.

None of the above trainers relied especially on brain maps when they first began using NFB. Some of them still do not use them. So, moving training locations was not an especially important consideration for them. Bill Scott (personal communication) differs from many people in that he trains with one electrode at C3 and the other at Fpz with eyes open and ignores the entire artifact. He claims that this clients still train well. At New Mind, we have tried it, and he is right. For more on this procedure, see the sample QEEG report in Chapter 4.

Early in the development of the field, most practitioners were using common protocols that seemed to work well with different disorders. New protocols were continually developed. An example is the Peniston protocol for treating alcoholism and addictions. The exact nature of the protocol was never clearly reported, but those who have spoken to Peniston personally indicate that they only up-trained 8-12 Hz at 01. Their equipment, at that time, did not have a means of training theta. Later, they added 8-12 Hz up with 4-7 up. The exact thresholds are unclear to this day. These latter sessions with PTSD used O2.

In the beginning, NFB involved a small group of practitioners at the ISNR and Futurehealth, Inc. It was very exciting to compare notes and discuss case histories. NFB is now larger, more complex and sophisticated. The use of QEEG is common and the technology behind expert systems like Val Brown's is very esoteric. The Othmer methodology has grown very complex as well. The addition of LENS and the fantastic claims regarding Z-score training confuse the picture even more.

Tool Box Approach

All of these methods are very effective and provide important pieces of the puzzle. That is why we promote the idea of the clinical tool box. The question new practitioners entering the field need to answer is, "Which protocols work best for me and my clients?" There is no replicated research to date that clearly indicates one method as being better than another. Practitioners may have to buy a couple pieces of equipment and try out a couple of methods before they feel confident in their clinical applications of the technology. Attending just one workshop or reading one book will not launch a practitioner confidently into a career in NFB. That being said, Joel Lubar (personal communication) has put together a valuable list of protocols found in the existing research literature that he has found to be effective.

Table 10 on page 125 shows these protocol guidelines. This list is integrated into the protocol suggestion section of the New Mind MiniQ report system.

The Othmers have developed a system in which they take baselines at C4, Cz, and C3. Based on symptoms, they determine how to train each side of the brain. They have developed a sophisticated decision tree based on their extensive clinical experience and the findings of their affiliate clinics. In the most simple terms, they tend to speed up the left side or slow down the right side of the brain or do a little of both at each session. Consequently, for someone with depression they would most likely do beta training on the left side at C3. For anxiety they would more likely do SMR training at C4. This approach is still widely used and has been expanded by many trainers and clinicians.

Sue Othmer has pretty much abandoned this approach for a new bipolar montage method that involves a comprehensive EEG inhibit with a select moving window of enhancement. This has recently evolved into training frequencies below 1 Hz, sometimes down as far as .01 Hz. This method is sometimes called sub-delta training. Practitioners definitely need to take several of her workshops to master this approach.

Table 10: Protocols Supported by Peer Reviewed Journal Articles
(from Joel Lubar—2001 Workshop ISNR)

Disorder	10-20 Site	Number of Sessions	Protocol Enhance Inhibit	
ADD	Pz age 7-9	30-50	16-20 Hz	4-8 Hz
	Cz age 10-15	30-50	16-20 Hz	6-10 Hz
	Fz age 16-25	30-50	16-22 Hz	6-10 Hz
	Fz age 26-50	30-50	16-24 Hz	6-10 Hz
ADHD	Cz or C3	20-30	12-15 Hz	4-8 Hz Or 6-9 Hz
Seizure disorder	Cz or C3	30+	12-15 Hz	4-8 Hz Or 6-9 Hz
Diseidetic dyslexia	P3 or P5	30+	beta	4-8 Hz Or 6-10 Hz
Disphonetic dyslexia	F3 or F5	30+	beta	4-8 Hz Or 6-10 Hz
Tourette's syndrome Tic disorders	Cz or C3	30+	SMR	4-8 HZ
Anxiety disorders	P4 or O2	Varies	Alpha 8-12	beta 15-24
Depression	F3 & F4	20+	alpha F4 Or train ratio of alpha F4 to F3	alpha F3
OCD	F4 or P4, P6	20+	Alpha 8-12	beta 15-24
Insomnia (sleep onset)	Cz or Fz	Varies	theta 4-7	beta 15-24

In Table 11: Early Othmer Protocols, on page 126, locate the symptom and find the protocol to use listed at the top of the column. Sue Othmer would usually inhibit 2-7 and 23-38 or some similar high and low range in addition to up-training one of the frequencies below. For instance "C3 Beta Up" might include 2-7 inhibit, 16-19 enhancement, 23-38 inhibit.

Valdeane Brown began in a very similar way. Val, however, began training both sides at the same time: beta on the left and SMR on the right. In addition, he would suppress both the low frequencies and high frequencies, which he usually found to be a source of problems. He saw this method as a sort of remedial work to stabilize the brain and normalize circadian cycles. Once this was accomplished, his next step or "period" of training involved something very similar to alpha-theta training. Finally, he finished up with a protocol that focused on two specific frequency ranges that he found especially valuable in enhancing transcendent insight and spiritual awareness.

Unlike many other clinicians, Val includes an explicit spiritual component in his model of training. This situation is not surprising, since most of clients seem to wrestle with spiritual issues toward the end of their training cycles—even when the topic isn't mentioned. According to the literature, many psychologists and counselors find themselves forced to deal with this dimension with their clients in the later stages of psychotherapy. Clearly it is an emerging trend and is further discussed in the section on alpha-theta training.

Table 11: Early Othmer Protocols

C3 Beta Up Theta Down Turning Up the CNS	Cz Beta	Cz SMR	C4 SMR Up Theta Down Turning Down the CNS
Inattentive	Bruxism	Anxiety	Impulsivity
Difficulty staying asleep	Night terrors	Panic	Bipolar
Social anxiety	Narcolepsy	OCD	Restless leg
Depression		Tics	Sleep apnea
Eating disorders		Onset insomnia	Poor social skills
Poor word fluency		Restless sleep	Migraine
Poor reading comprehension		Seizure	Aggressive and manipulative
Math problems		TBI	Rushes through work
PMS		Spasticity	
Memory problems			
Explosive rage			

- Val has multiple tones going at the same time and feeding back to his clients. He maintains that this is not a problem because NFB is not an especially conscious process. We also may use as many as three tones at the same time, but we find that we must follow certain rules with this procedure. For instance, the tones should at the very least harmonize with each other, as dissonance tends to be a punishment rather than reinforcement for most people (Z-score training presently uses one tone, scale of tones, or image to train 240 variables over four channels in the domains of phase, coherence, symmetry, and power).

- Bilaterally suppress 3 & 5 Hz, 8-13 Hz and 23-38 Hz. Simultaneously, augment C4 SMR and C3 beta. Symptom resolution through re-establishing circadian cycles.

- Bilaterally suppress 3 & 5 Hz and 23-38 Hz. Bilaterally augment alpha. Self-integration through profound relaxation.

- Bilaterally suppress 3 & 5 Hz, 8-13 Hz and 23-38 Hz. Cycle between bilaterally augmenting 19-23 Hz and bilaterally augmenting 38-42 Hz. Spiritual transformation through transcending multi-focal awareness and deconstructive presence.

- Table 12: The Period 3 Approach (Val Brown), below, shows this.

- Bilaterally suppress 3 & 5 Hz, 8-13 Hz and 23-38 Hz. Simultaneously, augment C4 SMR and C3 beta. Symptom resolution through re-establishing circadian cycles.

- Bilaterally suppress 3 & 5 Hz and 23-38 Hz. Bilaterally augment alpha. Self-integration through profound relaxation.

- Bilaterally suppress 3 & 5 Hz, 8-13 Hz and 23-38 Hz. Cycle between bilaterally augmenting 19-23 Hz and bilaterally augmenting 38-42 Hz. Spiritual transformation through transcending multi-focal awareness and deconstructive presence.

Table 12: The Period 3 Approach (Val Brown)

C4	C3	Purpose
3-5 down 8-13 down 23-38 down 13-15 (SMR) up	3-5 down 8-13 down 23-38 down 20-30 up	Symptom resolution through re-establishing circadian cycles
3-5 down 23-38 down 9-11 up	3-5 down 23-38 down 9-11 up	Self-integration through profound relaxation
3-5 down 8-13 down 23-38 down Cycle between: 19-23 up & 38-42 up	3-5 down 8-13 down 23-38 down Cycle between: 19-23 up & 38-42 up	Spiritual transformation through transcending multi-focal awareness and deconstructive presence

At present, Val has begun working at a whole new level, integrating his past efforts with a more refined approach with his NeuroCare Pro® system. He poses an interesting challenge to the whole field. Can an expert system like his be used safely and effectively by the general public? Even Siegfried Othmer (personal communication) has begun to talk about a home trainer in every living room. Val may have to show through thorough research that his theories are correct and his system safe enough for mass consumption before it is accepted.

Table 13: Single-Channel Monopolar and Bipolar Protocols

Disorder Protocol	10-20 Site	Number of Sessions	Protocol Enhance	Inhibit
Alpha training	P4 or Cz	20-40	9-11 Hz	4-7 Hz 20-30 Hz
Alpha-theta	Pz	30+	5-8 8-11	1-5 13-30
Seizure	Cz	30-40+	13-15	1-4 20-30

Table 14: Two Channel Monopolar and Bipolar Protocols

Disorder	10-20 Site Channel 1, 2	Number of Sessions	Protocol Enhance	Inhibit
General	C3 Fz C4 Pz	30-40	15-20 9-11	2-7 12-15
General	F3 C4 Pz	30-40	15-20 9-11	2-7 12-15

Table 15: New Mind Protocols (Eyes-Closed)

Purpose	10-20 Site	Number of Sessions	Enhance	Inhibit
Relaxation	Pz	Alpha-theta	5-8 8-11	2-5 15-30
Relaxation	Pz		8-12 70%	8-12 20%
Relaxation				
Relaxation	Pz	Hi amp alpha 10-12 Hi amp alpha 8-10	8-10 13-15	10-12 8-10
Relaxation	P4		9-11	
Relaxation	P4		9-11	2-7 20-30
Relaxation	P4		9-11	15-30
Relaxation	P4		8-10	
Depression	F3			8-12
	F4		8-12	

Table 16: New Mind Protocols (Eyes Open)

10-20 Site	Conditions	Enhance	Inhibit
C3 Fpz	Attentional	15-20 20-30	2-7
C3 Fpz		15-20	20-30
C3 Fpz		15-20	8-12 20-30
C3 F3		15-20	20-30
Fz		15-30	2-7
F3		15-30	8-12
C4 Pz	Relaxation	9-11	
C4 Pz	Anxiety	9-11	15-30
C4 Pz		9-11	20-30
C4 Pz		13-15 (SMR)	2-7 20-30
C4 Pz		13-15	8-12 20-30
Pz	Relaxation	13-15	2-7
Pz	Anxiety	13-15	20-30
Pz	Hi amp alpha is 10-12 Hz	13-15	8-10
Pz	Hi amp alpha is 8-10 Hz	9-11	12-15

Table 17: Additional Protocols

Purpose	10-20 Site	Number of Sessions	Protocol Enhance	Inhibit
Seizure	Cz	30-40+	13-15 20-30	2-7
Pain	T3 T4	30-40	13-15	
TBI	T3 T4	30-40+	12-15	1-3

TRAINING BY QUADRANT

For many years, we have been talking about quadrant training rules and what training is possible in each quadrant. John Demos (personal communication) has found this a valuable teaching concept as well. When you try to choose a protocol for training, the choice will often be limited by rules governing each quadrant. Suppose a client has too little alpha and you want to up-train it. The quadrant rules say you can't train alpha in the left front; it is not a great idea for the left back quadrant either. You would be better off training alpha on the right side and in most cases the right posterior is best. Beta, on the contrary, is best trained up in the left frontal quadrant.

Below is a chart for quadrant rules, so that if you do a MiniQ assessment you have something to guide you in protocol selection. For instance, you can train alpha down in quadrant A, but not alpha up. You can train beta up, but not beta down. If beta is too high in the left front, you might want to train alpha up on the right instead of beta down.

Diagram 46: Training Quadrants

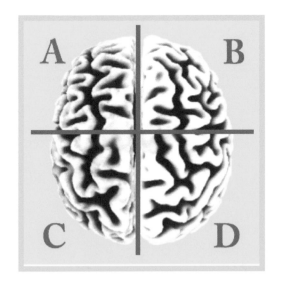

A: Alpha down, beta up, theta down, delta down

B: Alpha up, beta down, theta down, delta down

C: Theta down, delta down

D: Alpha up, beta down, delta down

THE PROTOCOL DECISION TREE

After doing a MiniQ assessment or QEEG—both of which are fairly common methods of assessment these days—you will find that there are several possible protocols you could try to remedy the problem. (See Peter van Dusen, John Demos, EEG Spectrum, Jon Anderson, Bob Gurnee, or Richard Soutar workshops for assistance.)

When difficulties arise, you need to decide the best protocol with which to begin and how long you should try it until you change it. To help with these decisions, we developed the Protocol Decision Tree. The rationale behind the Protocol Decision Tree evolved out of Richard Soutar's staff meetings at New Mind clinics over a decade. So, it came from "in-the-trenches experience" working with brain maps and a very wide variety of disorders and ethnic populations. New Mind Center has had offices in Phoenix, Shreveport, Atlanta, and Jacksonville, so the client population has been quite varied. New Mind Center records even show that there is a demographic difference in the types of depression that typically show up in a NFB office in the west coast versus the east coast.

The Protocol Decision Tree also provides clear steps to take once you have decided on the beginning protocol. If you can't make up your mind which protocol is best, then call for a consultation with someone with more experience. Once you start, you'll find that the method guides you quite clearly. Generally, you begin in one location and try different component bands. Then you move to a nearby site to train off site. If you are still not getting good results, try the next best location and frequency.

For example, if you have too much beta in the posterior region, you may initially try to train it down at Pz. If the beta does not train down easily, but the alpha goes up or the client becomes more anxious from the beta down-training, you may want to try and train the alpha up (the brain gave you a hint about what it might be willing to do). If you train alpha up and things go well, but beta does not go down, you might consider moving to P4 nearby, as that is an area that usually responds well to alpha up-training (see Diagram 46: Training Quadrants, page 129). When you train at P4, you might see alpha going up, beta coming down on its own, and the client feeling much better in the next session.

People often ask how long to try a protocol before they should switch to another. Our experience has been that some kind of change in client symptoms should occur within five sessions. Obviously, exceptions exist. If a client has a bad reaction, you should stop using that protocol right away.

THE COMMON THREAD

We find that a common thread exists between all these approaches. Rather than encourage just one or the other, we try to establish some basic principles to guide protocol development and implementation. Since New Mind Center has access to multiple databases, which we use on all of our clients, we have been able to watch for patterns of disorder and implement different protocol approaches developed by various experts to see what difference in effectiveness they might have.

We have found them all fairly equivalent in results. Some, however, do seem to work better with certain individuals than others. It will clearly take years of research to determine exactly why. Unfortunately, no one has begun that research process in a formal manner.

During a brain map analysis of the E. Roy John databases (personal experience and observation derived from a decade of teaching others), it is easy to be misled if you don't look closely at the numbers and morphology. Jay Gunkleman (personal observation) also exhorts everyone to focus on this information in all of his workshops. This process can lead to a sort of electronic phrenology.[25] It is very important to analyze exactly what specific frequencies are deviant/off norm. The advent of the Thatcher and Hudspeth (personal observation) databases made this analysis somewhat easier with the development of one-Hertz bins. These tools allow us to look at each frequency band individually, see how it is distributed across the scalp, and determine whether it is outside the normal expected range.

We have found that a pattern exists in most of the disorders where the lower and/or higher frequencies become enhanced and the mid-frequencies become suppressed. Other variations may be a suppression of lower frequencies or a suppression of higher frequencies. The goal is to train in a manner toward normalizing the spectral distribution. Jay Gunkelman (in workshops and multiple discussions at every ISNR meeting from 2000-2008) calls this process "shaping the EEG." Interestingly enough, Valdeane Brown's protocols appear to do just that in a general shotgun manner. Adam Crane's (Crane & Soutar, 2000) general theory of NFB also fits roughly into this category. The Othmers (personal communication) are also inhibiting higher and lower frequencies and up-training the middle frequencies. In fact, all practitioners are doing a version of this method because it reflects how the brain works. Once you take your baselines, you should look for patterns that deviate from the normal distributions. If there is a trend in which alpha increases at C3 so that it is higher than C4, we need to either down-train alpha on the left or increase it on the right.

One last item to keep in mind as you are training: If you are reviewing the session as it progresses, the review should show in Hz (with eyes closed) alpha, theta, delta, and beta. With eyes-open training, the review should show in Hz delta, theta, alpha, beta.

Note: With BrainMaster,® you can create a review screen and monitor separate waves as the session progresses.

SIDE EFFECTS OF NEUROFEEDBACK

As with many treatments, whether drug or otherwise, NFB also has the potential to create side effects during or after a session. Below are a few areas to remember:

---

[25] Phrenology is a defunct field of study, once considered a science, in which the personality traits of a person were determined by "reading" bumps and fissures in the skull (http://en.wikipedia.org/wiki/Phrenology) 01/19/09.

- Watch out for anxiety, irritability, increased physiological activity/vitals, sleep disturbance, agitation, nausea, headaches, mood elevations, general discomfort.
- Slow cortical potential training at T3 T4 (Othmer) should be used for theta down-training only, as the temporal lobes are the least regulated part of the brain and most open to destabilization.
- Alpha-theta training can trigger trauma episodes and dissociation.
- Training beta down in the posterior may create anxiety.
- Training alpha down on the right may create anxiety.
- Sensitivity to drugs can also create reactions to NFB.
- Doing NFB can also result in iatrogenic effects.

The terms *iatrogenesis* and *iatrogenic artifact* refer to inadvertent <u>adverse effects</u> or <u>complications</u> caused by or resulting from <u>medical</u> treatment or advice. In addition to harmful consequences of actions by physicians, iatrogenesis can also refer to actions by other healthcare professionals, such as <u>psychologists</u>, therapists, <u>pharmacists</u>, <u>nurses</u>, <u>dentists</u>, and others. Iatrogenesis is not restricted to conventional medicine and can also result from <u>complementary and alternative medicine</u> treatment.[26] Cory Hammond (2008) has addressed iatrogenic effects from NFB.

SUMMARY

Clinicians who rely entirely on QEEG claim they get excellent results training at the site that is deficient or excessive in some frequency range. That has not been entirely our experience. Instead, our experience indicates that the best pattern of training is often along the lines of what the Othmers, the Lubars, Valdeane Brown, and Margret Ayers (personal communication) have found. All of these clinicians start their training at the sensorimotor strip and move outward, although of late the Othmers are frequently starting at the temporal lobes. Unless our brain maps clearly indicate one simple area of trouble, we often begin our training at the motor strip. We have found that we get the fastest results with this strategy. We are beginning to use a bipolar montage with this location as well. Why the motor strip may be the most robust starting point is not well explained, although many solid theories have emerged.

Note: Many neurologists see the frontal areas of the brain as an extension of the motor strip and the parietal areas as an extension of the sensory strip in terms of structure and function. This perspective makes the sensorimotor strip the structural-functional center of the cortex even though it is not the executive area. Consequently, its influence over thalamic function may be greater than that of other areas due to higher densities of primary systems innervation. Training at the sensorimotor strip also has the advantage of reduced artifact.

For those starting out in the present environment, Z-score training or using an automated protocol output such as the New Mind Database system may be the best, easiest, and most reliable solution. These approaches provide specific guidance and built-in controls with respect to protocol selection. As you gain knowledge and skill, you can branch out into more innovative protocols.

---

[26] http://en.wikipedia.org/wiki/Iatrogenesis 03/15/2010

When equipment problems occur, the value of your equipment decisions is immediately evident. Having quick and reliable service departments with competent service technicians is crucial. It also helps to have an extra backup machine. Richard once had to get an appointment with one manufacturer's service department, which took several days. They were very nice people, but it took him over six months to solve the problem. This hassle included shipping equipment back and forth and what seemed like endless phone calls. If Richard had only had one NFB unit, he would have had to stop doing NFB for those six months. Luckily, Richard had a background in electronics. Otherwise, he is not sure he would have had the patience to go the distance with this manufacturer and fix the problem. This situation can become a nightmare for clinicians who are not technically oriented.

Before you buy:

- Ask other clinicians about the service department of the companies you may be dealing with.
- Check to see how long they have been in business and their track record.
- Go to a conference or visit their offices and try out their equipment in real time.

Note: Many clinicians who did not test equipment or see it in action before they purchased it wish they had done so before purchasing.

Also, remember that machines are often built around the manufacturer's theoretical perspective with respect to EEG. Few, if any, pieces of equipment can do everything. Therefore, you should plan to buy at least two different pieces of equipment and make sure they do different, yet complementary tasks. This will expand your training capabilities and make room for changes in your technique as you grow.

When it comes time to set your equipment up for the first time, be prepared to have patience. We have never purchased a piece of equipment that did not require much time and attention before it was up and running in a clinically useful manner. Every machine has its quirks and it takes time to learn them. It is best to practice on yourself for a while until you get all the kinks worked out. We recommend a headset phone for this process, as it requires two hands to operate most equipment.

Note: Some programs are not happy unless they have exactly the right computer. We have built computers to specs just to avoid the "which computer is right" game.

REVIEW QUESTIONS

1) What differentiates a monopolar from a bipolar protocol?

2) Why is training by quadrants important?

3) Which conditioning type best describes neurofeedback?

4) What are common reference points in neurofeedback?

5) What are common grounds when using neurofeedback?

CHAPTER 7: EVALUATION OF PROGRESS

THE CLINICAL PROGRESSION

Having your own protocols and established procedures makes a difference in how well your practice operates. We have developed a pattern of client management that has been very successful. Many clinicians come to our practice to shadow our staff members and get a feel for how the office flows, what the paperwork looks like, and how the practice operates. Sometimes this process is crucial for clinicians to put together all they have learned at workshops, so that they can develop their own practices with confidence. Other practitioners intuitively grasp how they want to incorporate neurofeedback and integrate it easily.

OUR PROCEDURES

When patients first contact us, we invite them in for an initial interview, so we can get acquainted and explain NFB to them. It usually takes an hour to discuss their problem, explain NFB, demonstrate a program, and discuss fees and schedules. Once they have decided to commit to doing sessions, they fill out the paperwork including history, client rights and privileges, and financial responsibilities. As mentioned in Chapter Five, providing a brochure that describes QEEG, NFB, homework, lifestyle changes, and expectations is a valuable way to assist patients and help them remember all that is discussed in the initial interview.

During the next appointment, clients have a brain map or QEEG and a TOVA, and fill out the Beck Depression Inventory or the Interactive Self Inventory. We may also do some memory testing and a Heart Math evaluation. These tests cover testing of the three primary frontal networks related to memory (dorsolateral), attention (anterior cingulate), and socio-emotional processing (orbital-frontal).

During the following appointment, we review the test results and correlate them with the client's symptoms. We list the symptoms we want to track, such as headaches, insomnia, low energy, etc., and then explain the protocol we will be using. In addition, we use the brain map to explain the process we will follow to obtain the desired results.

KEEPING RECORDS

Keeping good records is crucial to effective training, and may be a requirement of state regulations, licensure, accreditation requirements, etc. We take eyes-open or eyes-closed baselines at each session. These procedures often involve a 1- or 2-minute sample. We also do baselines to check asymmetry and pre/post- Rolandic baselines at regular intervals. Frequently, we chart client symptom changes and match them to changes in protocols to evaluate the effectiveness of our protocols (see C: Forms, page 175) We keep hard copies of these records in client files rather than rely upon computer-based client management programs, which may experience serious problems. This method also allows us to enter data into a general database management program like Excel, which can be later transferred to SPSS or SASS. This way, our data analysis is not limited. If you are unfamiliar with these programs, most grad students are good with them and can be hired at very reasonable fees to do the work for you. More and more NFB programs provide better statistical output that requires the use of other programs unless you are interested in doing research. Appendix D Forms, page 175, shows New Mind's Training Session Report form to use an example, but it is best to create your own form based on your office needs.

In addition, we record changes in client symptoms and have a checklist as part of the Training Session Report. A sample checklist is located on page 179. This checklist insures that the staff covers each important item. This information is placed in a folder with the bio-diagnostic, treatment plan, and protocol worksheet (see Appendix D for all the forms). Recently, we have begun to move this symptom evaluation to the internet, so clients can answer these questions from home. This process can be done by any clinician through the New Mind Maps site: www.newmindmaps.com.

IMPLEMENTING PROTOCOLS

Once you have done an intake interview with your client and established his or her problems, you will use these symptoms as your subjective indicators of progress. If they have insomnia, headaches, and low motivation, then you will watch how these indicators vary during the training process. Specific symptoms can be added to the Symptom Checklist on page 179. You will be trying to correlate these indicators or symptoms with the QEEG or initial multiple-site analysis. You have done your analysis and decided on a protocol. Now it is time to begin training.

We usually do three 10-minute trials during training except when we do alpha-theta. In that case, we do as many 10-minute trials as we can before the hour is up. We can usually get three 10-minute trials in within the hour. Most clients get tired by the third trial and show progressively worse results. With children, we will do either three 7-minute trials or four 5-minute trials, depending on their problems and their age. With experienced clients, we may do two 15-minute trials if it fits their protocol.

At the outset of each session, we go over the client's list of indicators to see if any changes have occurred. We may ask the client about other indicators as well. On the top left of our Training Session Report on page 179 is a list of common indicators that are reviewed each visit. Clients often begin to sleep better and dream more. They may find themselves less likely to respond in their usual way when their "buttons are pushed." It is always a good idea to ask questions and probe for things that have changed. Often, important changes occur without clients' knowledge; they may fail to mention them or to note their importance.

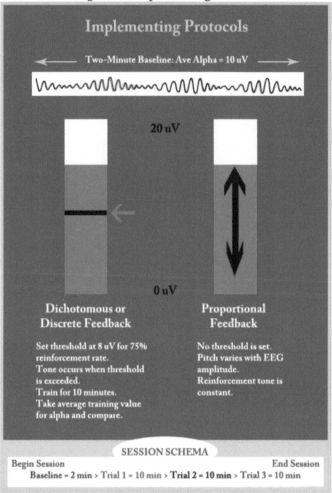

Having hooked our client up, we take a 1- to 3-minute baseline at the beginning of each session (see Diagram 47, above). A new baseline is important because baselines vary somewhat from day to day due to ultradian rhythms,[27] amount of sleep, diet, level of anxiety, mood, and so forth. One of Robert Thatcher's technicians told me they found the EEG to be highest during the noon time period for most people, so it makes sense to try and train most people at the same time each day to avoid distortions due to these effects. Individuals usually stay within a certain range, however. Most literature says that it takes several minutes to get a good theta baseline for research purposes; however, we have found that 2 minutes is adequate for clinical work.

We then set dichotomous thresholds based on the baselines of that day. If alpha is 8μV and we want to set a threshold for enhancement, then we set the threshold at 2μV below that point, at

---

[27] Ultradian rhythm: A biological rhythm with an ultra-short period and very high frequency–e.g., heartbeat, breath.

6μV. If we wish to inhibit alpha, we set the threshold 2μV above that point, at 10μV. This usually results in an 80% or better reinforcement rate. We call it "The 2μV Rule." It works with most equipment, except BrainMaster.® When using BrainMaster,® you can watch the BrainMaster® rate of reinforcement on the fly and adjust it while training (see Diagram 48, below). This method is not always possible with other equipment that cannot be adjusted during training.

Diagram 48: Neurofeedback Session Review Screen (BrainMaster Technologies)

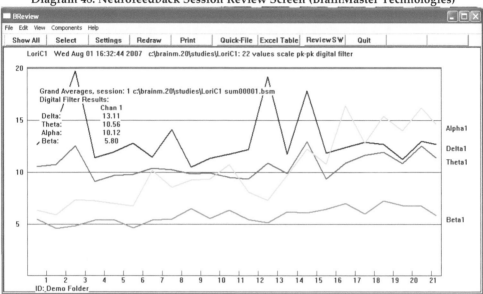

At the end of each trial we record their averages for each frequency that we are training. Often, we carefully watch other frequencies. For example, you may be training beta down, but also watch to see if alpha goes up and theta goes up or down. Compare the averages of each component band between each trial to see if the client is moving toward a normative distribution.

Note: You need to know if the average alpha on each trial is higher or lower than the baseline.

Keep in mind:

- A .5μV increase over baseline is significant.
- A 1μV increase is very good.
- A 2μV or more increase is excellent.

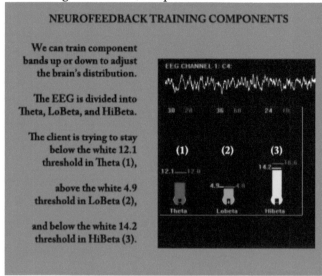

Sometimes the client's alpha may not increase, but the beta will decrease. This change is significant as well. It is important to watch all the component bands to look for changes. Some programs provide training graphs to show you all the subtle changes during training. These programs provide a more effective evaluation of training efforts.

If the client is able to attain or exceed his or her baseline on the frequency in which the client is training during a trial in the first five sessions on a regular basis, then we feel confident the client will make good progress in the next fifteen or so sessions.

Note: If clients fail to exceed baseline during these first trials, then we find it will often take them well over 30 sessions to achieve good results. We have come to this invaluable conclusion after years of clinical experience and analysis of client performance. This information is very helpful in offering clients an idea of their expected progress over the coming sessions.

PLASTICITY

Plasticity[28] may be the most valuable measure of progress in terms of EEG information available without a brain map. We have found that most clients with disorders have a very rigid EEG, so that when they up-train one frequency, all the other frequencies go up as well in proportion to the one on which they are focused. As clients get better, they are able to up-train the frequency of interest with less of an effect on other frequencies. If they are up-training alpha, then the other frequencies should go down in relationship to alpha. Other frequencies may go up in amplitude

---

[28] Plasticity is the lifelong ability of the brain to reorganize neural pathways based on new experiences.

somewhat, but their ratio to alpha should be less. So, whether we are training one or two frequencies at a time, we always carefully watch the other frequencies. The same goes for down-training a frequency band.

DOING WHAT WORKS

When choosing a protocol, you may try several variations at the outset to see which one is most effective. If a client has too much central beta, then you may try down-training beta, or up-training alpha—whichever provides the best result. In this case, a brain map may reveal that the client's amplitude in beta is three to four standard deviations above the database mean. This indicates that the client's EEG may be putting out all that it can in every frequency and that up-training is almost impossible. Without the brain map, you would not know that this is the case, but by trying different variants of the same protocol you can see that down-training beta works best.

Once you decide on a protocol, you can probably try it for five sessions or so to see if the results are consistently good. You should watch for changes in client indicators. If results are not emerging, then you might consider another location and protocol.

Note: Remember that it takes more energy for the brain to produce high frequencies than low frequencies. Consequently, small changes in beta have more significance than changes in lower frequencies.

TRAINING OFF SITE

When the initial multiple baseline analysis is done, you may find an area that is particularly abnormal. In attempting to run the appropriate protocol for several sessions, you may also find that the client is not making any progress moving above baseline. (This situation is explained in the latest research in TBI and computer simulations of what we know about hub and network systems.) This situation is fairly common. To make more rapid progress, you may want to train at the next nearest site where the abnormality is a little lower. Often clients can initially do better at this site, and then when good progress is achieved, you can move back to the worse area and get better results.

THE BRAIN'S WISDOM

When training, it is valuable to watch the interaction between individuals and their brains. The more entrenched and intense the disorder, the less control they have over their brains. You can immediately see the disconnection in the way they train. The brain seems to have a will of its own, and it is a great struggle. Fighting this tendency directly is often a futile effort.

When abnormal amplitude is present, it usually increases and decreases in a cycle very much like a swell in the ocean. We have often watched frustrated clients fight against the peaks as they occur when they are trying to down-train a particular frequency band. We try to get them to focus their energy on the dips when they are down-training and the peaks when they are up-training. We compare it to surfing—when you catch the wave and ride it.

Clients train better on some days than on other days. Often, they become too concerned with the numbers and become frustrated or discouraged. When this discouragement happens, we tell our clients that it is the effort that counts and that working hard at it on a bad day is just as important as on a good day—perhaps even more so (more research is needed on this situation). We also remind them of the progress they have made so far.

FREQUENCY OF TRAINING

The question clients ask is "How often should I come in?" because the answer directly affects their schedules and their pocketbooks. Many clients are disconcerted when they hear, "Twice a week at least." We have trained some people once a week; they do make progress, but it is much slower. This area is another place where we need more research. Training three times a week is even better. On the other hand, you should discourage clients from training every day. Often changes may come too quickly for them, and they end up on an emotional roller coaster that is overwhelming.

It is helpful to view brainwave training as exercising the brain. When you overwork a muscle in the gym, it will cramp on you and be sore the next day. It is better to work it gently and give it frequent rests. The same applies to the brain. By giving it a day or two of rest in between workouts, you give the client's brain time for integration and growth. We know of no research to support this, but many of the clinicians with whom we have talked have adopted the same position. On the other hand, Bill Scott's (personal communication) research suggests that this is not really necessary with regard to training attentional problems, so clinicians should not consider it an actual training limitation. In addition, most clients cannot afford to train every day and don't have the time. Making such a commitment can overwhelm them and cause them to give up early in the training.

The 30-Sessions Myth

We always hear stories of how people were cured in 15 sessions or 30 sessions. Some of the most competent NFB specialists we speak with at conferences frequently do not find this miraculous recovery rate consistently accurate. There are two main reasons for this:

1. The concept of cure should not be considered applicable in biofeedback. We are not medical doctors and we don't cure diseases.

2. The amount a client "improves" depends on the measure of improvement used. There is no standard in the field, so we are comparing apples and oranges here.

Many long-term disorders take 60 or even 100 sessions to resolve, if you have high standards as a clinician and rigorous outcome measures. By promising a client significant results too quickly, you may be doing a disservice. Letting a client go prematurely may result in relapse. That is why we use objective measures to evaluate clients.

We have had an amazing recovery of function in many cases in as few as 15 sessions, but this is the exception. What we do experience is rapid improvement in symptoms in 10 or 15 sessions if the client is training well. However, we understand that this is often only the beginning of the client's full potential for recovery of mental order and function.

DROP OUTS

No matter how good you are or how effective your practice is, the time will come when a patient comes in for treatment, attends 10 sessions or so, and then drops out of treatment.

Examples

One patient we worked with was doing poorly in school. She was not promoted to the next grade. She began treatment in mid-summer and had trained for four sessions by the time she began school again in late summer. The teachers were amazed at how much better she was doing during the first few weeks of school. Her attention was better. Her grades improved. She was told that if she continued to do well, she would get promoted to the next grade by the Christmas holiday. She attended a total of eight sessions and then just stopped coming to treatment. When contacted, she said she was doing great, feeling better, and didn't feel the need to come back . . . objective achieved.

Another patient had nine sessions and wanted to be remapped because he was not feeling a sense of improvement. To honor his request, we conducted a second map, which in fact showed some improvement in several areas. Despite the findings, he did not return to treatment.

Possible Solutions

Some practitioners suggest selling prepaid NFB sessions in a package of 20 sessions. This encourages commitment at a fiscal level. The client is more likely to attend sessions as scheduled for 20 sessions. In many cases, this will result in both the practitioner and the client experiencing improvement.

There is no single best solution to the dilemma of patients who drop out of treatment or do not attend sessions on a regular basis. All of us need to be prepared for such and to come up with creative methods to encourage hesitant clients to continue in treatment.

EVALUATING PROGRESS

You should evaluate progress at every session by talking with clients about their subjective indicators and their present training levels. If progress is slow and you are around the twentieth session, you should take another brain map.

Using the New Mind protocol with two channels at the same time, some practitioners have had rapid changes occur (as fast as or faster than Z-score training) that require a map every 15 sessions or even more often. Interesting information will often show up. We have not often found major changes in amplitude baselines during training, and it can be discouraging to have clients focus on them. The brain map usually shows changes that cannot be found during training baselines. Our position is that in the absence of a brain map, the ongoing evaluation is the best measure of progress. After all, it is the symptoms that brought the client in, not his or her baselines.

Psychometric tests are especially valuable for evaluation. We usually use a Beck inventory for a client with issues regarding anxiety and depression. We find that this inventory correlates nicely with changes in the brain maps, as does the TOVA for clients with ADHD. These tests are fairly quick, inexpensive, and easy to administer, and they provide valuable information regarding changes. For individuals with short-term memory issues, we use the digit span section of the Wechsler Intelligence Scale for Children (WISC), which is also quick and easy to use.

These tests can be used repeatedly with good results and help greatly in objectively documenting client progress. Recently, we have begun to use components of the Memory Assessment Inventory (MAS) memory test to find out more details about memory problems if the client is suffering from TBI. Clients may quickly forget their progress and habituate to their new conditions. When the training is difficult, it is helpful to provide objective documentation of their progress.

Quite often, we will use a personality inventory on clients who make slow progress. Frequently, this option can save valuable time and money. PTSD can often mimic other disorders and clients will forget or minimize the importance of traumas in their lives. For example, we were treating one client for depression. She recovered from the depression quite well, but her marriage became worse. She started to exhibit new maladaptive behaviors. We thought she had a personality disorder, but we gave her a Personality Assessment Inventory (PAI) and found she had PTSD. When we began treating her for PTSD, her progress rapidly improved.

Note: Research indicates that tests are generally more accurate in evaluating for particular conditions than even the most seasoned clinicians. If you can't do the testing yourself, then refer the client to someone who can.

OUTSOURCING

We have a psychologist for testing, a neurologist for trauma and organic disorders, an M.D. for medical problems, a psychiatrist for medications, and a counselor who specializes in violent children. They are not in our office, but we refer clients to them all the time. We have found professionals who believe that what we are doing is important and are willing to work with our clients in the capacity we wish. As we work with our clients' doctors, etc., we try to provide them with information on NFB and meet them for lunch to get acquainted. As a result, we have built a reliable network for support that benefits all parties and makes it possible for us to provide the best service for our clients. We try to keep to our NFB specialty as much as possible. We find this makes the training far more effective.

ETHICS

Our field has an ethical standard that each of us must follow. The Biofeedback Certification Institute Alliance (BCIA) has a set of "Ethical Principles of Biofeedback." This can be located at: http://www.bcia.org/associations/5063/files/EthicalPrinciples.pdf.

It is important to read and comply with these standards. As you continue your practice, you may have a client who comes to you for treatment after having left another professional's practice. The client may even complain about the professional's practice from an ethical concern. Should this occur, first contact that professional to understand both sides of the problem.

For example, assume a practitioner is treating an adolescent who sustained a TBI from playing hockey. In this scenario, the practitioner informs the client that during the course of NFB treatment the client should refrain from playing hockey or any other sport that might result in another head injury, i.e., lacrosse, soccer, football, etc. However, the client, against the practitioner's advice, continues to play hockey and sustains another head injury. The practitioner then tells the client that NFB treatment will not continue while the client engages in activity with a high risk for head injury. Then the client walks out of that practitioner's office and tries another practitioner.

In this case, the first practitioner followed a protocol that he or she believes in. The next practitioner might tell the client that s/he will continue treatment, but that continuing in a sport that puts the client at risk for a subsequent TBI is not in his or her best interest. This is just one example of the ethical concerns we all face. As Cory Hammond (personal communication, February 5, 2009) notes:

> Personally, I'd consider it unethical not to inform them strongly that continued head injuries could do further damage and undo progress. But I don't refuse to continue seeing them, but I keep telling them stories as we're working about cases where people have continued risky behavior and we've seen the results.

Some of the more general concerns among seasoned clinicians include:

Scope of Practice

Does the state licensing board under which you are licensed provide for doing NFB under that license's scope of practice?

> Practitioners should know the laws of their individual state in reference to who is and who is not legally allowed to provide biofeedback, psychotherapy, and other health care related services. Laws in some states restrict the provision of some health care services such as biofeedback and psychotherapy to members of specific disciplines, and some do not allow licensed practitioners to supervise

unlicensed personnel in the provision of these restricted services. What do the relevant laws in your state say governing the provision of biofeedback, psychotherapy, and related services? It is critical that you know what the provisions of your state laws are. Colorado has licensing laws governing the practice of specific disciplines like psychology, social work, nursing, and physical therapy, but it allows unlicensed practitioners to register themselves as unlicensed psychotherapists and to provide such services as biofeedback.[29]

Claims about Training Outcomes

As noted above, it is important to be honest and clear with potential clients about the benefits and potential outcomes of NFB. All of us will eventually be faced with a difficult case where the patient's progress is slow, and the patient drops out or requires a higher number of NFB treatment sessions to achieve some benefit.

Educational Requirements for Members

This field is growing at a rapid pace. It seems that new science in the field of neuroscience is appearing every week. It is important to keep up with the discoveries, research, and general practice concerns when performing neurotherapy.

Professional Responsibility and Liability

Make sure you have insurance and that your insurance provider is aware of the elements of your practice. As noted above, make sure that doing NFB is within your scope of practice, and if need be, that you are practicing under the direct supervision of a qualified professional.

Continuing Education Requirements

It is important to keep up with current trends and the science within our field. If you become BCIA certified, you will be required to attend a specified number of hours of CEU trainings.

Standards of Practice

This is a part of our ethics, and all NFB practitioners should be aware of and follow the ethics for our field as outlined by BCIA. For more details on ethics visit BCIA at: http://www.bcia.org/associations/5063/files/EthicalPrinciples.pdf.

Advertising

As we have noted above and throughout this book, it is important that you do not advertise your work with false claims and information.

Licensure

Most manufacturers require that you be licensed in order to buy their equipment. To protect yourself, you should be licensed, and if you are not, you should be operating under the supervision of a licensed professional.

---

[29] http://bio-medical.com/news_display.cfm?mode=MUL&newsid=68

Mentoring

Mentoring is the best way to learn the principles and practice of QEEG and NFB. If you plan to be BCIA certified, you will be required to go through a formal mentoring process that is documented.

As regards the use of technicians with inadequate training, and who are not fully supervised by licensed people:

If you work in a practice, clinic, or hospital setting where you have technicians working under you, it is important that they have adequate training, guidance, and ongoing supervision. In our practice, we require our technicians to engage in a specified number of hours of observation of our work, followed by a specified number of hours of practice under our direct supervision. They are required to complete readings and manuals and then pass a competency exam. Once they are practicing as technicians, they still need to be under your direct supervision.

It is important not to conduct the sale, rental or lease of home training units without ongoing supervision of the use of those units; supervision includes structuring things so that there is assurance that the home training units are not being used by parents on people other than their own children.

Do not bill insurance, Medicare, or Medicaid for biofeedback/neurofeedback or QEEG services by representing them as psychotherapy or psychological testing. Be sure to use the appropriate codes that have been created already for these services.

Suggested Reading on Ethics

There are two excellent articles in the *Journal of Neurotherapy* authored by Cory Hammond that address ethics and standards of practice in our field. These are listed below:

Hammond, D., Walker, J., Hoffman, D., Lubar, J., Trudeau, D., Gurnee, R., & Horvat, J. (2004). Standards for the use of quantitative electroencephalography (QEEG) in neurofeedback: A position paper of the International Society for Neuronal Regulation. *Journal of Neurotherapy, 8*(1), 5-27.

Hammond, C., & Kirk, L (2008). First do no harm: Adverse effects and the need for practice standards in neurofeedback. *Journal of Neurotherapy, 12*(1), 79-88.

In addition, there are articles published by Seb Striefel (1989, 1995) on the topic of ethics and biofeedback that practitioners should review before sitting for the BCIA test or beginning their NFB practices.

REVIEW QUESTIONS

50) How many sessions on average should be run before expecting to see progress with a client?

51) If a client comes to your practice and complains about the ethics of a previous professional, what should you do?

52) Why is tracking a client's symptoms on a weekly basis important?

53) After starting NFB, when should you consider remapping a client using QEEG?

54) Should we advise patients that neurofeedback is mostly experimental?

Chapter 8: Alpha-theta Training

Alpha-theta training is very similar to plain alpha training, but with some important exceptions. Alpha-theta training is a more passive process than other forms of feedback. Its goal is to achieve a temporary and profound liminal (in-between) state between sleeping and waking. In this state, the mind can be deeply probed, instructed, and directed or conditioned. This training is highly effective with a variety of disorders, especially anxiety, and has often been referred to as slow-wave training to distinguish it from fast-wave training such as the Othmers originally employed.

Background

Alpha-theta first came to the public's attention through the publication of a series of journal articles authored by Eugene Peniston and Paul Kulkosky (1989) of the Menninger Clinic in Topeka, Kansas. Since that time, quite a few well-designed and executed replications have been published. In spite of this, a great deal of myth and misunderstanding continues to surround the protocol and how it should be implemented. In a conversation with Paul Kulkosky (personal communication), Richard has found that their original goal, to a large extent, was to up-train alpha in alcoholics who had too little of it present.

Much of the following background has been lost in the evolution of this protocol, but it is worth understanding. Elmer Green, a biophysicist, became involved in pioneering EEG training. He originally performed extensive alpha training followed by several weeks of theta training. His theory was that the initial extensive alpha training would allow individuals to maintain awareness longer than usual when placed in theta states of consciousness. As a consequence of this process, many of the individuals he worked with were having profound altered-state experiences including many that mimicked near-death experiences.

Gene Peniston was very impressed with Green's workshops and decided to try alpha combined with theta training on resident alcoholics; some accounts indicate that he got the idea while training himself with the protocol. Peniston formulated a unique combination of therapies that included NFB. He emphasized that NFB was only one component of his experiment and should not be considered the only important component. This statement was in response to many professionals who had concluded that NFB was the most important component, since it was the most innovative feature of the design, and the design was so successful in its outcome.

The original experiment involved placing an electrode at O1 on the occipital cortex and providing alpha feedback for a 30-minute session. Individuals were left alone to train in a dimly lit room. Theta was a questionable component.

Peniston (1989) appears to have set the alpha threshold at baseline and the theta threshold at an arbitrary 10 microvolts below the alpha baseline. The procedure was done five days a week for a total of 28 days. After each session, the experimenters asked the subjects what they experienced. However, the experimenters reportedly did not do extensive processing with them. The subjects were residents in the institution and may have been engaged in other group or individual counseling activities that were not reported.

The methods section is quite unclear about many details (Lowe & McDowall, 1992). At least one other researcher who attempted to replicate the study recently reported at an ISNR meeting that he found the original article insufficient in detail for replication and felt that this insufficiency contributed significantly to his failure to find the same results. Going back to Elmer Green's (1977) original writings regarding the subject, we find that his goal was to induce theta in the left occipital cortex and that he felt electrode placement was crucial.

In addition to the EEG training itself, some pre-training exercises were involved including relaxation exercises and hand-warming exercises. The hand-warming exercises involved attaching a thermistor (thermometer) to one hand and practicing raising hand temperature. Some research indicates that there is a correlation between theta production and hand-warming exercises. Peniston (1989) trained prospective clients in visualization, temperature training, rhythmic breathing, and autogenic training before engaging in alpha-theta training.

RECENT RESEARCH

More recent literature on the topic and workshops that we have attended have described interesting variants of this original approach. Like so many other forms of feedback, the techniques have become rigid and ritualized as if they contain some kind of magic. However, little attention is given to the rationale underlying the process. Many practitioners presently do this type of training at Pz, P3, and even Cz. Literature from Nancy White's early workshops (personal communication) documents this shift in electrode placement. An interesting crossover phenomenon has also begun to dominate the procedure.

The crossover phenomenon involves a point in the training when subjects begin to experience higher levels of theta than alpha. As individuals train in alpha, they often become drowsy and their alpha frequency slows and drops in amplitude, while theta amplitude theoretically increases. At a certain point, theta becomes higher than alpha. This occurrence indicates the production of hypnagogic [30] or hypnopompic images. These images reportedly hold key information that needs to be integrated by the individuals. Post-session interviews with clients focus on bringing these issues to the foreground of their awareness, so they can process them. Consequently, trainers tend to count crossovers and hyper-focus on this occurrence as an indicator of successful training.

Recent research on this topic indicates that there is not a direct correlation between crossovers and these images. However, if you include spontaneous visualizations, then there is an increased correlation. Either way, it may be dangerous to conclude that individuals are repressing material merely because they are not demonstrating crossovers.

---

[30] A hypnagogic image is a dreamlike image, often vivid and resembling a hallucination, experienced by a person in the transition state from wakefulness to sleep.

Other problems arise with this approach as well. Many individuals have baselines with theta already higher than alpha. This scenario makes it impossible to have a crossover unless you train them in alpha alone. You could attempt to up-train them until their baselines changed; however, baselines may not change that significantly after many sessions even though there is significant improvement in presenting problems. With these individuals, we find that up-training alpha alone results in hypnagogic images, spontaneous significant visualizations, and abreactions. Thus, you need to be prepared to address these experiences when they occur as a result of alpha-theta training as described below.

Many variations regarding threshold settings exist as well. Settings for alpha vary between 50% and 80%. Settings for theta vary between 20% and 60%. This situation is interesting because ratio strain should occur below 70% reinforcement rates. This scenario means that reinforcement is so low that the operant behavior is poorly elicited. In other words, you are no longer using operant conditioning. A 10% to 40% reinforcement rate may be useful, however, in that the theta tone may occur during crossover and heighten the subject's awareness while in theta. Again, the underlying theory is that the client needs to produce more alpha initially to enter a state of drowsiness and reverie in order to get into the theta state.

The consequences of alpha-theta training can be very uncomfortable for clients. Abreaction is common, especially in clients with PTSD. Clients may cry, twitch, become restless, moan, and so forth. The common method of dealing with this situation is to leave them alone as much as possible and get them to continue to focus on training. Many practitioners believe these experiences generate a type of systematic desensitization. When the session ends, it is important to discuss what the client experienced, but it is not necessary to do an in-depth analysis. It is a good idea to be sure that PTSD clients have access to a counselor, so they can process some of the material that surfaces. For those without PTSD, post-session periods of moodiness or anxiety that can be uncomfortable may occur.

Note: Clients need monitoring in this area and reassurance that the discomfort will pass in a few days.

Most practitioners have their clients do a 10-minute session of SMR enhancement with theta down-training to get clients clear and to help them integrate material that emerges in the session. We have also used SMR after visualization sessions and find it very effective for the same reason. Some practitioners, like Bill Scott (2002), inhibit 3-5 Hz to reduce abreactions and report that this strategy is effective and does not seem to interfere with the training. Scott came up with this idea when he was training some Native Americans who kept falling asleep during the sessions. He originally thought he could train delta down to keep them awake. It not only helped keep them awake, but their abreactions began to reduce significantly in intensity and frequency.

Abreactions can occur outside the office; it is important to warn your clients of this possibility. Some people with histories of severe trauma are physically and emotionally incapacitated for days. Prepare them for this possibility and have them come in or contact their counselors if this occurs. In addition, make sure their counselors know what is going on, so they can assist you—especially if you are not their primary therapist. At New Mind, we have clients sign a form (see

Appendix D, page 175) that explains the possible side effects of the therapy and basic client responsibilities.

Many practitioners such as Martin Wuttke (personal communication) insist that clients do preliminary SMR training or deal with abnormal brainwave activity before engaging in alpha-theta training. He also trains individuals in diaphragmatic rhythmic breathing as well. Alpha-theta training is often contraindicated for individuals with ADHD, schizophrenia, epilepsy, stroke, and head trauma. Bill Scott (2005) reports that he trains individuals from all these categories, but does fast-wave training with them first until their TOVAs show normal results. We have found that individuals with high theta have all they can handle in terms of abreactions with alpha training alone.

If you plan to work with individuals with addictions, it is important to get them to stop "using" for the process to be successful. They should also be attending a support group of some kind. The recommended training is daily for 30 days. If they "use" during the training period, they may experience flu-like symptoms or have severe hangovers.

For example, one client who failed to go to meetings went ahead and drank his beer, but found that it tasted funny and did not have the expected effect. Consequently, he went out and bought a bottle of Jack Daniels to do the job. Needless to say, he dropped out of the training.

SESSION PROGRESSION

Bill Scott (2005) perfected several methods while performing his research. The following information is taken from that research.

Prior to doing alpha-theta training, it is helpful to get a complete history and a TOVA. If the TOVA indicates any attentional problems, these problems should be addressed first. The TOVA is used as a guide to design the protocol.

Usually, beta 16-20 Hz is up-trained on the left side with inhibits on 23-38 Hz and 2-7 Hz. SMR is up-trained on the right side with the same inhibits. Scott trains one side (hemisphere) at a time during the sessions. He trains more on the side of the brain that appears weakest on the TOVA. If a client performs poorly on omissions, then Scott will train more on the left side. If the client scores poorly on commissions, then Scott will train more on the right side. The montage he uses is C3-Fpz for left-side training and C4-Pz for right-side training. Amplitudes tend to be low because he uses bipolar montages. A great deal of artifact occurs due to eye blinks when training on the left side.

Note: Originally, we were skeptical of the value of training at all with the level of artifact we experienced, but Scott encouraged us to ignore it. To our surprise, clients improved greatly in spite of the artifact.

One of the most surprising things to come out of Bill Scott's (2005) research regards training session frequency. Scott found he could not only train people every day, but even twice a day. This frequency means he was able to normalize an individual's TOVA in 14 or 15 days!

Remediation of attentional problems can be very rapid. Of course, for most people this can be a burden rather than a help. At New Mind we still tend to train people two or three times a week, but are willing to do more intensive training. We do have some people who are training every day.

Once a client's score on the TOVA falls into normal range, it is time to make preparations for the deep states training. Some form of relaxation training is very helpful. We have used finger temperature, skin conductivity response (SCR—also known as SCL, EDR, and GSR), HeartMath® or heart rate variability training, and breath work. At this point we have found that breath work is most effective for us. This training tends to accelerate clients' learning curves when it comes to moving into deep states during NFB. For breath work, we use Respirate®.

Another important area of preparation is visualization. We have professionally made relaxation and visualization CDs created by Barbara Soutar[31], which were designed specifically for this purpose. These visualizations are integrated with audio visual entrainment (AVE) to assist individuals movement from state to state. We find the entrainment accelerates the learning process for most individuals, but we also use the CDs effectively without entrainment. Many people are not used to actively visualizing scenes and need some initial practice. The CDs provide that practice. In addition, since more salient issues tend to surface during the relaxation and visualization practice, clients become more aware of the issues that they need to work on during alpha-theta training.

It is important for clients to use a visualization that is consistent with their goals. Goals can be solutions to problems, abstinence, performance, and insights into behavior. Usually, trainers instruct clients to focus on their visualizations at the beginning of the sessions and then to let go and focus on the NFB.

This method can be a good approach, but it is not the only way to use visualization. You should not be afraid to innovate with the process, if you feel intuitively that an adjustment could be effective in assisting change. Once clients have practiced visualization and have decided on a specific visualization to use, they are ready to begin formal training.

After clients are hooked up and the filters are set with the correct frequencies and thresholds, they begin their visualizations, and then focus on the tones. Inevitably, most people start to experience an alpha drop out as they drift into deeper states. They also begin to lose self-awareness. At a certain point, the theta grows higher than the alpha. When this occurs, they begin to experience more theta reinforcement than alpha. This point is a good time to tweak the threshold by increasing or decreasing it, so that they are actively getting theta reinforcement.

---

[31] Available online at www.newmindmaps.com

Clients will experience periodic resurgences of alpha that bring them back into greater self-awareness and then slide back into theta. The beta inhibit will assist those clients with anxiety from getting overly aroused when this shift occurs. Clients tend to swing back and forth like this until they begin to drift into sleep. At this point, delta will begin to rise in amplitude. As your client nods off, you can note the delta level and readjust it, so a sound of some kind will rouse the client. We use an alarm clock sound in one of our programs that goes off when delta goes above its baseline value. Elmer Green (personal communication) used to tie one of the client's fingers to a mercury switch and have the client hold his or her arm up by resting the elbow on the chair. When the client drifted off, the arm would drop and the mercury switch would set off a doorbell. When clients experience a complete cycle like this, you will know how to set their thresholds exactly. Scott tends to sit through the session and "ride" the thresholds the whole time.

At New Mind, we tend to just let clients train alone, although we constantly check on them to make sure they are doing well and that the electrodes have not fallen off. Clients will swing back and forth between full awareness and sleep. Over a series of several sessions, they will get better and better at balancing in a deep state between sleep and waking. This deep state is really the goal of the training.

Diagram 50: Thresholds, page 154, shows the different frequencies and how to set the thresholds as discussed. Client EEG averages tend to look like the pattern shown. After training with their eyes closed for a few minutes, the pattern tends to shift to the pattern shown in at the bottom (see Diagram 51: Threshold after Eyes-Closed, page 154). Delta tends to be highest, with theta next highest and alpha the lowest. Clients will shift back and forth from the top pattern to the bottom pattern as they train. It is during these shifts that they will have crossovers.

Crossovers vary in length and importance, as previously mentioned. They tend to begin somewhere between the fifth and the tenth sessions. The longer the cross-over, the less likely clients are to recall any associated images and the more likely they are to drift into sleep. The images may or may not have pertinence to them at the time. Our most seasoned clients can drop into long crossovers without going into sleep and remain there for five or ten minutes at a time. This may or may not be valuable, depending on the goal of the training.

When clients finish the session, it is a good idea to review their experiences, both physical sensations and psychological events. Frequently, clients will realize their success while they are outside of the office. Some clients have no hypnagogic experiences at all, but instead have intense and sometimes lucid dreams. These dreams may sometimes hold the key to fundamental issues.

Diagram 50: Thresholds

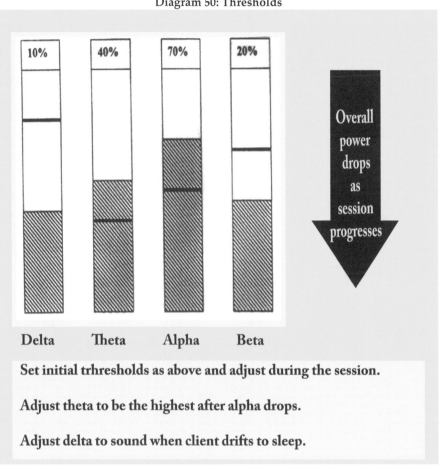

Set initial trhresholds as above and adjust during the session.

Adjust theta to be the highest after alpha drops.

Adjust delta to sound when client drifts to sleep.

Diagram 51: Threshold after Eyes-Closed

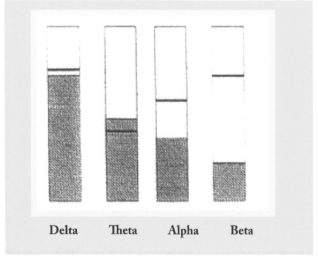

REVIEW QUESTIONS

55) What is the value of alpha-theta training?

56) What creates crossover?

57) What is a hypnagogic image?

CHAPTER 9: AUDIO VISUAL ENTRAINMENT (AVE)

DEFINITION OF AVE

MindAlive defines AVE as follows:

> AVE is a technique that provides light pulses complimented by sound at specific frequencies, tones and beats, via a portable audio-visual entrainment (light and sound therapy) device. Using flashes of lights and pulses of tones, AVE safely guides the brain into various brainwave patterns. . . .
>
> This stimulus connects with the brain at the specified frequency that can be programmed into the control device by the user. Typical brainwave frequencies are described as alpha, beta, theta and delta. Each of these frequencies has a corresponding brain behavior associated with them. Alpha and theta are associated with a dreamy, languid state of mind and less focus, beta is associated with a highly focused mind set, and delta is associated with a sleep state. . . .
>
> Based on the desired change in behavior, the light and sound pulses enhance the production of the specific brainwave frequency targeting the desired behavior(s), settles down an agitated mind, increases cerebral blood flow, and increases the metabolism of glucose in the brain for improved neuronal function. All of this activity adds up to improved mental performance.[32]

A key objective of entrainment is to produce a dissociative state, which is similar to a near sleeplike state of deep relaxation. When AVE is used, the dissociative or relaxed state can be observed by noticing deeper, diaphragmatic breathing than before the use of the device. Blood flow to the frontal lobe will also improve. The relaxed feeling is facilitated by beneficial neurotransmitters being released into the brain.

AVE has many benefits for adult and adolescent users. The regenerative process has proven useful for many of the emotional and physical challenges that our stressful lives present to us daily. These conditions include anxiety, depression, insomnia, migraines, PMS, high blood pressure, and chronic fatigue, along with improved attention, learning, and reduction in symptoms of ADD and ADHD. Those adults and students who have experienced problems with getting the proper sleep will also find AVE to be beneficial.

RESEARCHING AVE

Initially, many practitioners were suspicious of entrainment, discounted its possible value, and were overly concerned regarding possible side effects such as seizure. Unfortunately, almost all of these concerns were based on uninformed opinion and hearsay. No one read the research regarding this subject. As it turns out, research on photic stimulation is considerable and goes

---

[32] Adapted from: http://www.mindalive.com/index.htm and David Siever

back to the first half of the twentieth century. A few people like Tom Budzynski (personal communication) were using it quite extensively early in the game and were well acquainted with its potential. When Richard first purchased a unit at the Futurehealth Conference in the mid 1990s, fairly important key players in the field whispered to him about the dangers inherent in this technology. Since that time, the technology has become more widely used, and workshops held on the topic are more heavily attended.

Fortunately Richard met Dave Siever, who set up a group entrainment experience for those in attendance at the conference. It was astonishing. Richard found out later that Julian Isaacs (personal communication) was doing group sessions with entrainment at Esalen as well. At New Mind, we used the device on ourselves and were able to explain away all the mythology.

After a while, we employed it in conjunction with EEG on healthy golfers who were interested in peak performance. The results were very impressive. Over time, we began to use it regularly with our clients. It became a common part of our protocols because we found that it facilitated the EEG sessions greatly when clients were just starting out. As a stand-alone technology, we found it could stop migraines, reduce pain from fibromyalgia and RSD, almost eliminate TMJ, improve sleep, and increase mental clarity, among other things.

Since that time, Richard has completed considerable research with his client population and reported the results at ISNR. In addition, he has held workshops on the topic. It is surprising to find out how many practitioners do not know about its value in EEG training. Fortunately, during the 2001 SNR meeting, the AVE panel (AVE is Dave Siever's term for entrainment) talked to a full house about entrainment. Later, Richard was stopped by many people who talked about how much they enjoyed the presentation and told him they planned to start using this technology more; thus, we wrote this chapter on a most important topic. There is greater detail on it Dave Siever's (1999) book, *The Rediscovery of Audio-visual Entrainment Technology*, available from the Mind Alive website[33]. We recommend that you read this book from cover to cover before using entrainment.

In an effort to determine some AVE training guidelines, Richard reviewed much pertinent research with the help of a grad student working on her Ph.D. on entrainment effects. Her goal was to extract essential features of various findings that could be operationalized in the clinical setting. Casting these findings into a group of axioms with regard to the clinical use of AVE and consequently testing their potential value as hypotheses for research seemed an essential step in evaluating this developing technology. This review is noted further in this chapter.

As mentioned, we have found that the research supports what we have discovered on our own about the use of entrainment. We employ it like training wheels during the initial sessions of EEG training. We find that individuals can learn to produce EEG above or below baseline faster when initially assisted by entrainment.

---

[33] http://www.mindalive.com/2_0/Rediscovery.htm

Note: Over time, however, the entrainment begins to interfere with NFB training instead of enhancing it. At this point, we stop the use of entrainment.

USING AVE

At New Mind, our usual pattern of initial EEG training begins with a baseline. We then train using the appropriate protocol for 10 minutes. Next, we train the same frequency with AVE, using the glasses only. During this process, the client gets audio feedback from the NFB equipment regarding his or her performance. On the third trial, we train without AVE again. We are only using the visual component of AVE without headphones, but it works quite well in conjunction with the NFB. We have found from experience that the audio component does not contribute significantly to the process, and the headphones can introduce artifact. As a rule, clients generally do much better when assisted by visual entrainment while doing the NFB. They almost always do better on the third trial.

It is very important to use sinusoidal or near-sinusoidal light pulses to get true entrainment. Only a few products on the market provide this feature. The square-wave light pattern that many manufacturers offer is less effective at generating entrainment; it produces entrainment in unwanted frequencies and carries a greater risk of inducing seizure activity in individuals prone to seizure. White light is also the safest to use. Red light is more irritating to individuals with instabilities. Make sure you question prospective clients thoroughly regarding seizure history. Be sure to ask them if they have or of anyone in their family has a history of seizure.

Note: We have learned from experience to avoid using AVE on clients with abnormal EEGs due to their experiences of exposure to toxic substances that have generated toxic encephalopathy.

In addition, we have found that entraining the frequency you plan to up-train with the NFB works well for up-training, but down-training is more complex. The best approach to down-training is to train just off the harmonic above or below the frequency you plan to down-train. For instance

- To down-train 9 Hz, run the entrainment device at 19 Hz.
- To down-train 6 Hz, run the entrainment device at 13 Hz.
- To down-train 18 Hz, run the entrainment device at 10 Hz.

Entrainment is great for client management as well. When clients come in sleep deprived, give them a 20-minute entrainment session to put them into a sleep-like dissociative state and refresh them. They can usually do better on their training afterward. Ten Hertz usually does the job quite well and is safe for most clients. For kids with ADHD, a 10-minute session of 14 Hz with their favorite music will calm them down. Clients who are also jarred from the traffic on their way to your office can benefit from a few minutes of AVE before you begin the NFB trials. Be sure to take your baseline first, as the entrainment may alter it somewhat.

With some clients, such as those with fibromyalgia, you may want to rent them a unit to take home to use as needed. This practice is very effective at reducing their pain and can accelerate their progress in the office.

We have used AVE very successfully in the home setting with kids with ADHD. It is easy and enjoyable for the kids to use and can make a big difference in their day. It also helps calm the nerves of their parents, if we have the parents use it as well.

Overall we think you will find this technology a highly useful and cost effective addition to your practice. Be sure to read up on it, take some workshops, and research your equipment purchase carefully.

Much of the early research regarding entrainment focused on establishing the existence of entrainment and exploring the essential features of the basic phenomena. Kawaguchi et al. (1993) noted that these early studies focused on the existence of the driving response, responsivety, latency of response (cortical resistance to entrainment), and variability of response.

EARLY RESEARCH

Loomis, Harvey, and Hobart (1936) found that individuals with strong alpha rhythms had a narrow frequency range in which entrainment took place, whereas those individuals with low alpha had a much wider frequency range of entrainment. This discovery was repeatedly explored over the next several decades. James Toman (1941) followed up this research with findings that replicated the earlier work.

Walter and Walter (1949) determined that photic stimulation can cause EEG patterns to match the frequency of the driving stimulus. Gastaut and Hunter (1950), on the other hand, concluded that a difference probably exists between spontaneous brain rhythms and photic driven rhythms and consequently developed another major theme to be pursued in future research. Garoutte et al. (1958) also found considerable variation in subjects regarding how well EEG binds to photic stimulation rhythms.

Barlow (1959) continued to investigate whether entrainment resulted in a change in natural EEG, or if the response occurred in special networks related to intrinsic EEG phenomena. After concluding that entrainment was actually taking place, he noted that the frequencies of entrainment did not generate mirror images in the EEG, and there could be a highly variable relationship between input and response. He theorized that both EEG and "sensory after discharge" occur in nonspecific systems to generate alpha, but that the two systems might still be separate. Tweel and Lunel (1965) also found that amplitude of EEG response was often independent of amplitude of stimulus, but response reflected input character in terms of amplitude and frequency. They also found that out-of-phase stimulation in both eyes produced cancellation effects.

Ulett (1957) reported on his own findings as well as provided summaries of many other interesting research efforts up to that time. In particular, he focused on susceptibility to entrainment in low and fast frequency ranges of anxiety-prone individuals. He found that the driving response fluctuated from day to day based on mood. There was a relationship examined between colors seen during photic driving, amount of movement perceived in eyes-closed patterns, and Rorschach responses, with rigid personalities exhibiting less of both colors and movement.

Some of his findings follow:

- Shifts in blood oxygen saturation had been reported to occur at specific frequencies.
- Photic stimulation could cause visual hallucinations related to past experiences along with irregular bursts of slow-wave activity.
- Specific frequencies could cause subjective dysphoria in some individuals.
- Specific frequencies could cause myoclonus or paroxysmal activity and could lower seizure thresholds.
- Photic shock was thought to be more effective and less destructive than regular shock therapy.
- Sleep deprivation increased myoclonic and paroxysmal responses to photic driving.
- Metabolic changes could alter responses to photic driving.

He even reported on research in which it was found that photic stimulation paired with sound can generate the same rhythm when the sound is played back. These findings suggest a multitude of confounds that can be present when experimenting with photic stimulation and that are not usually considered in more modern research. This evidence seriously calls into question the internal validity of many of these studies.

Deiter and Weinstein (1995) agreed that photic driving increased alpha beyond natural levels and acknowledged that theta produced altered states with hypnagogic phenomena. Iwahara et al. (1974) explored more complex aspects of the components of photic stimulation than had been previously considered. They found that the entrainment that occurred was the result of a combination of EEG, photic driving effect, and a blocking effect. The blocking effect resulted in a reduction in EEG amplitude due to the stimulus that was present, but was not usually considered. They felt this research supported the idea that the photic driving effect was a different phenomenon than just the increase in basic EEG activity and that the research supported earlier researchers who had concluded that it occurred in different circuits.

Townsend (1975) began exploring sinusoidal modulated light (SML) and determined that it is different than photic driving. SML is more specific in its action upon the EEG with less activity occurring outside the alpha range. The degree of entrainment at the cortex depends on the proximity of the driving stimulus frequency to the dominant alpha frequency. Entrainment also reduces frequency variability without appreciably altering morphology. The average evoked EEG response amplitude is highest at the dominant resident alpha frequency. He also concluded that the driving response occurs in other networks and alters natural EEG through this mechanism. Unfortunately, he and previous researchers fail to discuss what these networks might be, how they relate to natural EEG networks, and how they specifically alter EEG. The theory behind all this research was apparently not well developed.

159

Takahashi and Tsukahara (1976) experimented with colors and frequencies to determine what would be most likely to induce a seizure or photo-convulsive response. They determined that the color red in conjunction with 15 Hz was most likely to induce this phenomenon.

RECENT RESEARCH

Moving into later research, we find that brain imaging becomes more important and that there is a continued focus on physiology. Fox and Raichle (1985) reported that regional cerebral blood flow increased in the striate cortex by 28% due to photic stimulation. Mentis et al. (1997) reported that photic stimulation activates the frontal area of the brain. Diehle et al. (1998) found that significant cerebral blood flow increases due to photic stimulation.

Pigeau and Frame (1991) found that subjects with high amplitude alpha baselines showed best entrainment at frequencies closest to their spontaneous peak alpha frequencies. Low alpha baseline subjects, however, didn't appear dependent on this same phenomenon. Subjects with low amplitude alpha baselines, on the other hand, were more responsive across the alpha range and more responsive across all frequencies. The authors concluded their research with the theory that high and low alpha baselines may represent the degree of coupling between two different alpha sources in the cortex and subcortex. Strongly coupled thalamo-cortical connections could be reducing cortical activity, which shows up as high alpha with a strong spontaneous peak alpha frequency (lack of plasticity). Low-amplitude alpha may represent poor thalamo-cortical connections and less stable spontaneous peak alpha frequency. Of special interest is the neurophysiological theory proposed with regard to the phenomena studied, and the suggestion that the path of entrainment is through the lateral geniculate nucleus into the visual cortex via geniculo-calcarine radiation.

Kawaguchi et al. (1993) investigated inter- and intra- hemispheric synchrony and found that repetitive flashes enhance these phenomena, but they are not consistent during photic driving. They concluded that the lateral geniculate nucleus is the main player in setting up resonance between EEG and photic driving.

Patrick (1996) used AVE in place of NFB on ADD using EEG monitoring to confirm a client's ability to duplicate AVE experience (small group). Morse (1993) reported that AVE with tapes works better than AVE alone.

Rosenfeld et al. (1997), building especially on Pigeau and Frame (1992), found that high baseline alpha showed no entrainment at 10 Hz, and low baseline alpha showed transient entrainment (stopped when stimulus stopped). However, they were only able to explain 25% of the variance through baseline considerations. They further found that training just off the spontaneous peak alpha frequency tended to inhibit rather than enhance alpha production. They indicated that high alpha baseline subjects showed no entrainment at 22 Hz stimulation and that low alpha baseline subjects did show transient entrainment. Furthermore, beta entrainment also produced increased alpha in some individuals. They concluded that effects of entrainment cease once stimulus is terminated. They also agreed with previous researchers that no evidence showed what had been called "sensory after discharge" or entrained EEG and that spontaneous EEG arises from the same pathways. Lubar (1997, 1998) found in two studies that dominant alpha frequency training with AVE increased eyes-open beta and reduced delta. Budzynski (1999) performed a pilot study that indicated that AVE can shift dominant alpha frequency upward. Shealy (1990) reported that 10 Hz AVE increases serotonin levels by 20% and beta-endorphins by 14%. He found that the optimal session length is 20-30 minutes and that most people prefer violet light. He also reported that variable frequency is best for dealing with pain.

RESEARCH ON THE USE OF AVE WITH SPECIFIC DISORDERS

In addition to the impact photic stimulation has on physiological and psychological features associated with anxiety, other exploratory research efforts indicate it has considerable potential with a variety of other disorders.

Solomon (1985) found AVE to be effective with muscle-contraction headaches but not with migraines (small group study).

Anderson (1988) found it effective with migraines (small group study).

Norton (1997) found it useful for treating PMS (small group study).

Carter and Russell (1993) used it successfully with Learning Disorders.

Montgomery et al. (1994) used it successfully with closed head injury, aneurysms, and stroke.

Kumano et al. (1996) found it effective with depression in a highly criticized study (single case design). Cantor and Stevens (2009) on the other hand did a well designed small groups study that also should significant reductions in the symptoms associated with depression.

David Noton (1995, 1996) found that PMS symptoms were reduced by 50%.

Michael Joyce (1998) was successful using it with ADD, and D. J. Anderson (1989) regularly stopped migraines with AVE.

Tom Budzinski (2002) reported use of AVE in the case of an Alzheimers patient that appeared to show promise in slowing the progress of decline.

ADDITIONAL RESEARCH ON SPECIFIC DISORDERS

Many other case studies and small group studies have been reported at meetings, but not yet been published, including work by David Trudeau (SNR 1999) using 18 Hz AVE for 60 sessions with chronic fatigue syndrome.

Dave Siever (SNR 1999) reported on using AVE alpha and/or delta (n = 51) in a study with fibromyalgia in which he found good results and also another study with TMJ.

Some recent studies have also combined NFB and AVE:

161

Rozelle and Budzynski (1996) found that EEG-driven photic stimulation gives good results with stroke victims.

Carter and Russell (1993, 1997) found EEG-driven AVE to be effective with learning disorders.

PAST RESEARCH FINDINGS AND RULES OF ENTRAINMENT

It is clear from this research that AVE has considerable potential for a wide variety of disorders when used on its own; however, our main interest is whether it can be used to accelerate the NFB process. It seems to be effective in most of the same disorders as NFB and is likely to be of value in the same domains. This similarity causes us to consider the rules of entrainment when using it in conjunction with NFB. Where and when will it assist and where could it create problems? We constructed the following axioms of entrainment from the above research and our own clinical experience.

GENERAL FINDINGS OF AVE

- The effects of entrainment are highly variable between clients.
- The effects of entrainment vary between sessions.
- Individuals with low alpha baselines are most affected by entrainment with respect to EEG.
- Training is fairly effective across the spectrum.
- There are more effects outside the target frequency.
- Individuals with high alpha baselines are least affected by entrainment with respect to EEG.
- Training is most effective within the alpha range.
- Training is most effective at the dominant alpha frequency.
- Most of the entrainment effects with respect to EEG dissipate quickly after the entrainment device is shut off.
- There does appear to be some residual effect on beta amplitudes, which may last over 24 hours.
- Training next to a dominant frequency may cause cancellation effects.
- Training next to a dominant frequency may reduce EEG amplitude.
- AVE is more effective with music.
- Clients prefer violet light.
- It may be possible to classically condition a client's entrainment pattern to music.

SEIZURE CONCERNS

- AVE can temporarily enhance paroxysmal patterns in the EEG.
- Red frequencies are most likely to contribute to paroxysmal patterns.
- Frequencies over 15 Hz are likely to contribute to paroxysmal patterns.
- Square waves are more likely to contribute to paroxysmal patterns than sine waves.

MORPHOLOGY

- Square waves are more likely to generate harmonics.
- Sine waves are more specific in entrainment effects.

PHYSIOLOGY

- AVE reduces autonomic arousal.
- AVE increases frontal activity.
- AVE increases cerebral blood flow.
- High baseline alpha may indicate strongly coupled thalamo-cortical connections.
- Low baseline alpha may indicate poorly coupled thalamo-cortical connections.

PERSONALITY THEORY

- High responsivity to AVE in terms of color and movement may be correlated with flexible personality.
- Low responsivity to AVE in terms of color and movement may be correlated with rigid personality.
- The above axioms suggest a wide range of variables not reported or taken into account in most of the experimental designs executed so far.
- Case studies should carefully screen for all these factors.
  - Baseline Alpha Levels
    - mood
    - sleep patterns
    - metabolic changes
    - drugs taken
    - color of light used
    - type of wave pattern employed
    - personality profile
    - use of music

These factors constitute possible confounds with regard to both training and research and must be taken into consideration. The findings to date would seem to clearly emphasize the importance of regarding the brain not as a linear, passive system, but as a non-linear, reactive system with regard to outside stimuli. In the prevailing zeal to deal with objective phenomena, many seem to lose sight of the fact that EEG is coupled to very subjective phenomena. As stable as EEG phenomena may be with respect to averaged readings of power and frequency, it is still profoundly variable on an instantaneous basis and reflects subjective changes of state. These changes of state are linked to very subjective factors.

CLIENT REACTIVITY AND HISTORY: FURTHER CONFOUNDS

The research on AVE dealing with variables such as high and low alpha baselines does not as a rule extend its discussion into areas regarding what generates these differences in alpha baselines and appears to assume that they are normal variants. This is a dangerous assumption to maintain, as recent research suggests that high amplitude slow alpha and low amplitude fast alpha are often correlated with depression and anxiety disorders, respectively. This scenario is often the case even at a subclinical level.

The prevailing theory, of course, is that altering these baselines can reduce disorder and symptoms. However true this may be, the reverse should also be considered. Factors outside the clinic can cause symptoms to increase and generate client reactivity with respect to training. Internal environments are also likely to generate similar reactivity. In this sense, history often works through the reactive process to generate forces that mitigate training efforts. There *are* clients who do not respond to AVE or NFB.

De Goode et al (1972) indicated that expectation and cognitive set considerably influence alpha training. Lynch and Paskewitz (1971) noted that alpha only occurs in situations where subjects cease to attend to stimuli that normally block this activity, such as cognitive, somatic, emotional, and environmental events. Anxiety and depression both have ruminative features involving repetitive negative self-talk and related emotions. It may very well be these features that influence alpha baselines by engaging and occupying attentional networks.

We have had anxiety clients increase their alpha instantaneously by suspending their ruminative activities for a few moments. In similar situations, others have decreased their abnormally high amplitude alpha. In cases where individuals are so emotionally involved with internal ruminations that they cannot disengage, it is likely they will not do well with NFB. It is also likely that this applies to AVE. We have, however, observed variations in responsivity to NFB and AVE. Initially, many clients will generate higher amplitudes of alpha during AVE than during NFB. This suggests that attentional networks are influencing outcomes. Clients may be overusing active attentional networks during NFB, and consequently blocking alpha in their efforts to focus and concentrate on the stimulus tone.

THE ROLE OF ACTIVE AND PASSIVE ATTENTIONAL NETWORKS

Othmer et al. (2000) and Sterman (1996) observed that it may not be necessary that a conscious awareness of training take place for NFB effects to emerge. Margret Ayers (1999) worked with coma victims and supported this observation with empirical evidence as well. However, conscious efforts at training may not always be as successful as those efforts that bypass it. Kamiya (1979) discovered through experimental procedure that initial training of conscious individuals results frequently in an achieved average alpha that is less than baseline. Successive trials usually, but not always, result in training averages higher than baseline. This evidence suggests that conscious efforts alter the training pattern of NFB and vary its impact on subconscious operant processes. The variety of factors influencing this conscious effort may be quite large and could include a considerable number of interaction effects as well. In addition, the human unconscious response may also have considerable impact on training efficacy. The consequences for AVE may be similar as well.

An under-acknowledged assumption in previous decades is that EEG and NFB are being investigated in a passive system, i.e., the brain's response. Investigators have not clearly acknowledged that they are dealing with an active system that may respond in accordance with a number of variables so complex as to qualify as a non-linear chaotic system. Nunez and associates have recognized the non-linear characteristics present, but also have failed to recognize intentional and preconscious components driving that system. Whether the observer-subject is a consequence of the system or not has yet to be determined, but in either case the observer/subject surely constitutes a metasystem with its own unique characteristics.

This observer-subject system is often more reactive in a manner based on its history rather than immediate stimuli. This consideration calls for a different perspective than that which presently operates frequently in the EEG experimental environment. Although it is traditionally acknowledged in psychology that a subject's awareness of the purpose of an experiment can confound the internal validity of that experiment, those who have been conducting experiments with EEG, as well as clinical protocols, often assume that EEG operates independently from subject awareness. They assume that EEG could be consistently responsive to training independent of subjective factors known to influence it. The most curious part of this fact is that it even needs to be mentioned to psychologists engaged in research.

The implications of this consideration are that the presence of the subject's observer system can alter the nature of the object of experimentation, which in this case is the brain. The responses of the brain from this perspective constitute an active system with regard to the independent variable and can alter the definition, and consequently the effectiveness, of the independent variable, independent of the experimenter's definition. The subject's observer system can instantly alter the response pattern of the brain. It can anticipate, be proactive, and marshal resources to resist training or entrainment at a conscious or pre-conscious level of operation. This resistance process may be due to activities and responses of the observer that occur outside the clinical setting.

Our clinical experience indicates that subjects can frequently produce high levels of alpha EEG during entrainment while failing to produce similar results using NFB. Successive trials continue to produce this result, usually until baseline is achieved. Paradoxically, AVE at this point often proves to be less effective than NFB, with clients producing higher amplitudes without AVE. This also supports the notion that subjects are learning to use their attentional networks in such a way as to sustain attention, but not generate an alpha blocking effect. Active attentional shifts cause a reduction in average alpha as well as alpha amplitude, but sustained attention without active processing increases it. This outcome suggests the possibility that AVE engages a passive attentional network that the client eventually learns to employ with NFB as well over successive trials. At this point, clients not using AVE are able to more effectively use this network than with the AVE. Consequently, their NFB average amplitude is higher. What remains to be explained is why AVE amplitudes tend to decrease after this point.

Recent research literature provides evidence of an active and passive attentional system (Posner & Raichle, 1994). Active networks are employed to learn new skills and passive networks are engaged to execute those learned skills. Once alpha production has become an acquired skill, it

165

can be done with the passive network, which interferes less with alpha production because it does not involve as much active processing. The exact roles of the cingulate, globus palladus, and other neural structures have yet to be worked out. It is these networks, however, that would be the primary vehicles through which an observer-subject system would confound entrainment or NFB. More investigation regarding the relationship between EEG, attentional networks, and mood would further clarify existing relationships.

As previously mentioned, variance due to observer effect may be a consequence of immediate factors such as mood or rumination level as they affect EEG through attentional networks (assuming that these networks drive the RAS), or it may be due to social contextual factors extending beyond the immediate force of their influence. It may be impossible to clearly separate all of these variables. Lubar's (1999) observations regarding the influence of familial factors on the efficacy of training in the clinic further support this perspective. Trauma within the family system carries over into the clinical setting and emerges as resistance in the neural system to outside influences, including NFB and AVE. Similar effects are apparent in pharmacological interventions when dosage is increased to deal with increase in symptoms due to external stressors. The biological system has a preference for a particular neurochemical balance and resists efforts to shift that balance. The consequence of those efforts is often increased side effects.

Researchers such as E. Roy John (1988) have noticed immediate and dramatic shifts in QEEG configurations when cognitions commanding powerful emotional correlates temporarily generate QEEGs that mimic disorder. As we have said, our clients have demonstrated an ability to exert direct and immediate control over their EEG in such a manner as to apparently normalize their readings. The problem is that they cannot sustain that control over extended periods of time. They become distracted and fall back into automatic patterns of function. They have habituated to pathological network patterns.

CONCLUSION

Responses to NFB and AVE vary from day to day and trial to trial. This variance is due to a wide variety of extraneous variables frequently not accounted for in the literature. These variables may be a consequence of physiological factors or diurnal effects, or they may be a consequence of psychological factors such as cognitions and mood. The resistance to intervention is often active, with the brain responding robustly in the opposite direction of the training intentions. It is hypothesized that a preconscious system is proactively resisting intervention, preferring instead a state that has its origination in other social-psychological factors relating to the individual's history of observations and responses to the environment. These factors must be measured and accounted for if research efforts are to reflect accurately the effects of NFB and AVE interventions and if widely effective protocols are to be developed.

REFERENCES FOR AVE CHAPTER

Anderson, D.J. (1989). The treatment of migraine with variable frequency photo-stimulations. *Headache 29*, 154-155.

Ayers, Margaret E. (1999). Assessing and treating open head trauma, coma, and stroke using real-time digital EEG neurofeedback. In Evans JR, Abarbanel A (Ed.s), *Introduction to quantitative EEG and neurofeedback* (pp 204-220). San Diego: Academic Press.

Barlow, J. (1960) Rhythmic activity induced by photic stimulation in relation to intrinsic alpha activity of the brain in man. *Electroencephalography and Clinical Neurophysiology 12*, 317-326.

Budzynski, Thomas H. (1999). From EEG to neurofeedback. In J. R. Evans & A. Abarbanel (Eds.), *Quantitative EEG and neurofeedback* (pp. 66-76). New York: Academic Press.

Budzynski, T., Budzynski H., Jodry, J., Tang, H., Claypoole, K. (1999). Academic performance with photic stimulation and EDR feedback. *Journal of Neurotherapy 3*(3), 11-21.

Budzinski, T., Budzinski, H., Sherlin, L. (2002). Short and long term effects of audio visual stimulation (AVS) on an alzheimer's patient as documented by quantitative electroencephalography (QEEG) and low resolution electromagnetic brain tomography (LORETA) [Abstract]. *Journal of Neurotherapy, 6*(1), 69.

Cantor, D. S. & Stevens, E. (2009). QEEG correlates of auditory-visual entrainment treatment efficacy of refractory depression. Journal of neurotherapy: investigations in neuromodulation. *Neurofeedback and Applied Neuroscience, 13*(2), 100-108.

Carter, J. L., & Russell, H. L. (1993). A pilot investigation of auditory and visual entrainment of brainwave activity in learning-disabled boys. *Texas Researcher: Journal of the Texas Center for Educational Research*, 4, 65-73.

De Good, Douglas E., Elkin, Barry, Lessin, Steven, Valle, Ronald E. (1972). Expectancy influence on self-reported experience during alpha feedback training: subject and situational factors. *Applied Psychophysiology and Biofeedback 2*(2), 183-194.

Dieter, J. N. I., & Weinstein, J. A. (1995). The effects of variable frequency photo-stimulation goggles on EEG and subjective conscious state. *Journal of Mental Imagery, 19*, 77-90.

Diehl, B., Stodieck, R.G., Diehl, R.R., & Ringelstein, E.B. (1998). The photic driving EEG response and photoreactive cerebral blood flow in the posterior cerebral artery in controls and in patients with epilepsy. *Electroencephalography &Clinical Neurophysiology, 107* , 8-12.

Fox, P.T., & Raichle, M.E. (1985). Stimulus rate determines regional blood flow in striate cortex. *Annals of Neurology,17,* 303-305.

Garoutte, B and Aird, R.B. (1958). Studies on the cortical pacemakers: synchrony and asynchrony of bilaterally recorded alpha and beta activity. *Electroencephalography and Clinical Neurophysiology, 10,* 259-268.

Gastaut, H., Hunter, J. (1950). An experimental study of the mechanism of photic activation in idiopathic epilepsy. *Electroencephalography & Clinical Neurophysiology, 2,* 263-287.

John, E. R., Prichep, L. S., Fridman, J.,Easton, P. (1988). Neurometrics: computer assisted differential diagnosis of brain dysfunctions. *Science, 293,* 162-169.

Joyce, M., Siever, D. (2000). Audio-visual entrainment program as a treatment for behavior disorders in a school setting. *Journal of Neurotherapy, 4* (2), 9-25.

Kamiya, J. (1979). Autoregulation of the EEG alpha rhythm: A program for the study of consciosness. In: E. Peper, S. Ancoli, & M. Quinn, (Ed.s), *Mind body integration* (pp289-298). New York: Plenum Press.

Kawaguchi T., Jijiwa, H, and Watanabe, S. (1993). The dynamics of phase relationships of alpha waves during photic driving. *Electroencephalography and Clinical Neurophysiology 87*(3), 88-96.

Kumano, H., Horie, H., Shidara, T., Kuboki, T., Suematsu, H., & Yasushi, M. (1996). Treatment of a depressive disorder patient with EEG-driven photic stimulation. *Biofeedback and Self-Regulation, 21,* 323-334.

Loomis, AL, Harvey, EN, & Hobart, G. (1936). Electrical potentials of the human brain. *Journal ofnExperimental Psychology 19,* 249-279.

Lynch, James J., Paskewitz, (1971) David A. *Journal of Nervous and Mental Disease, 153*(3), 205-217.

Lubar, J.F. (1997). The effects of single session and multi-session audio-visual stimulation (AVS) at dominant alpha frequency and two times dominant alpha frequency on cortical EEG. Presented at the 5th Annual SSNR Meeting, Aspen, CO.

Lubar, J. (1998). An evaluation of the short-term and long-term effects of AVS (sound & light) on QEEG: Surprising findings. Presented at Futurehealth Conference on Brain Function, Modification & Training, Palm Springs, CA.

Lubar, J. F. & Judith Lubar (1999). Neurofeedback assesment and treatment for attention deficit/hyperactivity disorders. In James R.Evans & Andrew Abarbanel (Eds.), *Introduction to quantitative EEG and neurofeedback* (pp. 243-310). New York: Academic Press.

Mentis, M., Alexander, G., Grady, C., Horwitz, B., Krasuski, J., Pietrini, P., Strassburger, T., et. al. (1997). Frequency variation of a pattern-flash visual stimulus during PET differentially activates brain from the striate through frontal cortex. *Neuroimage, 5,* 116-128.

Montgomery, D. D., Ashley, E., Burns, W. J., & Russell, H. L. (1994). Clinical outcome of a single case study of EEG entrainment for closed head injury. *Proceedings from the Association for Applied Psychophysiology and Biofeedback*, 25, 82-83.

Morse, D. R. (1993). Brain wave synchronizers: A review of their stress reduction effects and clinical studies assessed by questionnaire, galvanic skin resistance, pulse rate, saliva, and electroencephalograph. *Stress Medicine*, 9, 111-126.

Noton, D. (1997). PMS, EEG, and photic stimulation. *Journal of Neurotherapy*, 2 (2), 8-13.

Patrick, G. J. (1996). Improved neuronal regulation in ADHD: An application of 15 sessions of photic-driven EEG neurotherapy. *Journal of Neurotherapy*, 1, 27-36.

Pigeau, R. A., & Frame, A. M. (1992). Steady-state visual evoked responses in high and low alpha subjects. *Electroencephalography and Clinical Neurophysiology/Evoked Potentials Section*, 84(2), 101-109.

Rozelle, G.R. & Budzynski, T.H. (1995). Neurotherapy for stroke rehabilitation: A case study. *Biofeedback and Self-Regulation*, 20, 211-228.

Rosenfeld, J.P., Reinhart, A., Srivastava, S. (1997). The effect of alpha (10 Hz) and beta (22 Hz) "entrainment" stimulation on the alpha and beta EEG bands: individual differences are critical to prediction of effects. *Applied Psychophysiology and Biofeedback* 22(1), 3-20.

Shealy, C. N., Cady, R. K., Cox, R. H., Liss, S., Clossen, W. & Culver Veehoff, D. (1990). *Brain wave synchronization (photo-stimulation) with the Shealy RelaxMate (TM).* Shealy Institute for Comprehensive Health Care: Springfield, MO.

Solomon, G. D. (1985). Slow wave photic stimulation in the treatment of headache-a preliminary study. *Headache*, 25, 444-446.

Sterman, Barry M.. (1996). Physiological origins and functional correlates of EEG rhythmic activities: implications for self-regulation. *Biofeedback and Self-Regulation*, 21(1), 3-33.

Takahasi, T., Tsukahara, Y. (1976). Influence of the colour on the photic convulsive response. *Electroencephalography and Clinical Neurophysiology 41,* 124-136

Toman, J. (1941). Flicker potentials and the alpha rhythm in man. *Journal of Neurophysiology 4,* 51-61.

Townsend, R. E., Lubin, A., & Naitoh, P. (1975). Stabilization of alpha frequency by sinusoidally modulated light. *Electroencephalography and Clinical Neurophysiology*, 39, 515-518.

Trudeau, D. (1999). A trial of 18 Hz audio-visual stimulation (AVS) on attention and concentration in chronic fatigue syndrome (CFS). Presented at the Society for Neuronal Regulation.

Tweel, L.H.,Lunel, H.F.E. Verduyn (1965). Human visual responses to sinusoidally modulated light. *Electroencephalography and Clinical Neurophysiology* , 8 (6), 587-598

Ulett, George A. (1957). Experience with photic stimulation in psychiatric research. *American Journal of Psychiatry 114*,127-133.

Walter, V.J., & Walter, W.G. (1949). The central effects of rhythmic sensory stimulation. *Electroencephalography &Clinical Neurophysiology, 1*, 57-86.

APPENDICES

APPENDIX A

SELECTED DISTRIBUTORS OF NEUROFEEDBACK EQUIPMENT & ACCESSORIES
(IN APLHABETICAL ORDER)

APPLIED NEUROSCIENCE, INC.

228 176th Terrace Drive
St. Petersburg, FL 33708
Phone: 727.244.0240
Fax: 727.392.1436
Website: http://www.appliedneuroscience.com/
E-Mail: QEEG@appliedneuroscience.com

BIO-MEDICAL INSTRUMENTS INC.

2387 East 8 Mile Road
Warren, MI 48091-2486
Toll Free: 800.521.4640
Phone: 586.756.5070
Fax: 586.756.9891
Website: http://bio-medical.com/
E-Mail: sales@bio-medical.com

BRAINMASTER TECHNOLOGIES, INC.

195 Willis Street
Bedford, OH 44146
Phone: 440.232.6000
FAX: 440.232.7171
Sales & Support: 440.232.7300
Website: www.brainmaster.com
E-Mail: sales@brainm.com

EEG INFO

6400 Canoga Ave, Suite 210
Woodland Hills, CA 91367
Phone: 818.456.5965
Toll Free: 866-334.7878
Fax: 818.373.1331
Website: http://www.eeginfo.com/

EEG SPECTRUM INTERNATIONAL, INC.

15400 SE 30th Place, Suite 205
Bellevue, WA 98007
Phone: 425.643.2495
Toll free: 800.400.0334
Fax: 425.644.7452
Website: http://www.eegspectrum.com/
E-Mail: evash@eegspectrum.com

ELECTRO-CAP, INTERNATIONAL

1011 W. Lexington Road
P.O. Box 87
Eaton, OH 45320
Phone: 800.527.2193
Fax: 937.456.7323
Website: http://www.electro-cap.com/
E-Mail: eci@electro-cap.com

MIND ALIVE, INC.

9008 - 51 Avenue
Edmonton, Alberta, Canada
T6E 5X4
Toll Free (within Canada and US): 800.661.6463
US: 780.465.6463
Fax: 780.461.9551
Website: http://www.mindalive.com/
E-mail: info@mindalive.com

OCHS LABS

503 S. Main Street
Sebastopol, CA 95472
Phone: 707.823.6225
Fax: 707.823.6266
Website: http://www.ochslabs.com/
E-Mail: cathywills@ochslabs.com

STENS BIOFEEDBACK - STENS CORPORATION

3020 Kerner Blvd., Suite D.
San Rafael, CA 94901
Toll Free 800.257.8367
Website: http://www.stens-biofeedback.com/
Email: http://www.stens-biofeedback.com/contactus

THOUGHT TECHNOLOGY, LTD.

USA
20 Gateway Drive
Plattsburgh, New York 12901
Toll Free: 800.361.3651
Fax: 514.489.8255

Canada
2180 Belgrave Avenue
Montreal, Quebec, Canada
H4A2L8
Phone: 514.489.8251
Website: http://www.thoughttechnology.com/
E-Mail: mail@thoughttechnology.com

WEAVER AND COMPANY

565 Nucla Way, Unit B
Aurora, CO 80011
Toll Free: 800.525.2130
Phone: 303.366.1804
Fax: 303.367.5118
Website: http://www.doweaver.com/
E-Mail: customerservice@doweaver.com

APPENDIX B

SELECTED TRAINERS IN NEUROFEEDBACK

RICHARD SOUTAR

New Mind Center
702 Macy Drive
Roswell, GA 30076
Phone: 678.516.5942
Website: http://www.mindmindcenter.com
E-Mail: drs@newmindcenter.com

JOHN DEMOS

Neurofeedback of South Vermont, LLC.
P.O. Box 325
Westminster, VT 05158
Phone: (802) 732-8060
Website: www.eegvermont.com
E-Mail: workshop@eegvermont.com

SIEGFRIED & SUE OTHMER - EEG INFO

6400 Canoga Ave., Suite 210
Woodland Hills, CA 91367
Phone: (818) 456-5965
Toll free: 866.334.7878
Fax: (818) 373-1331
Website: http://www.eegInfo.com

EEG SPECTRUM INTERNATIONAL, INC.

15400 SE 30th Place, Suite 205
Bellevue, WA 98007
Phone: 425.643.2495
Fax: 425.644.7452
Website: http://www.eegspectrum.com
E-Mail: info@eegspectrum

MICHAEL & LYNDA THOMPSON

The ADD Centre
50 Village Centre Place
Mississauga, ON
Canada, L4Z 1V9
Phone: 905-803-8066
            416.488.2233
Fax: 905-803-9061
Website: www.addcentre.com
E-Mail: addcentre@gmail.com

STRESS THERAPY SOLUTIONS

3401 Enterprise Parkway, Suite 340
Beachwood, OH 44122
Phone: 216.766.5707
Toll Free: 800.447.8052
Fax: 440.439.3015
Website:
http://www.stresstherapysolutions.com
E-Mail: stsinc@pantek.com

JON ANDERSON

Stens Biofeedback - Stens Corporation
3020 Kerner Blvd., Suite D.
San Rafael, CA 94901
Toll Free: 800.257.8367
Website: http://www.stens-biofeedback.com
E-Mail: stephen@stens-biofeedback.ccsend.com

Appendix C

Selected QEEG Databases

NxLink

NYU Medical Center Shool of Medicine
Brain Research Laboratory
Website: http://www.nyu.edu/brl/research/qeeg_database.html

NeuroGuide

Applied Neurosciences, Inc
Website: http://www.appliedneuroscience.com

SKIL

Sterman Kaiser Imaging Labs
Website: http://wwwskiltopo.com

NeuroRep

The Brain Resource International Database

Brain Resource Company
Website: http://www.brainresource.com

Institute of the Human Brain

HBIMed Brain Diagnostics
Website: http://www.hbimed.com

APPENDIX D: FORMS

NEW MIND NEUROFEEDBACK CENTER
PHYSIOLOGICAL HISTORY QUESTIONNAIRE

Have you experienced any of the following symptoms?

Place a number (for frequency) at the beginning of the item, and then place a letter (for severity) at the end of each item.

1=rarely	A=unbearable
2=sometimes	B=very unpleasant
3=often	C=unpleasant
4=very often	D=mild
5=all of the time	E=very mild

Example: _I_ Back pain _E_

_____Abdominal bloating _____

_____Headaches _____

_____Abdominal pain _____

_____Always sickly _____

_____Amnesia _____

_____Anxiety attacks _____

_____Aphonia (loss of voice above a whisper) _____

_____Back pain _____

_____Bulimia _____

_____Burning pains in rectum, vagina, or mouth _____

_____Chest pains _____

_____Constipation _____

_____Diarrhea _____

_____Dizziness _____

_____Dysmenorrhea (painful menstruation) _____

_____Dysmenorrhea-other _____

_____Dyspareunia (painful sexual intercourse) _____

_____Dysuria (painful urination) _____

_____Excessive menstrual bleeding _____

_____Extremity pain _____

_____Fainting spells _____

_____Fatigue _____

_____Fits or convulsions _____

_____Food intolerances _____

_____Frigidity (absence of orgasm) _____

_____Had to quit working because felt bad _____

_____Heart palpitations _____

_____Insomnia _____

_____Joint pain _____

_____Labored breathing _____

_____Lump in throat _____

_____Menstrual irregularity _____

_____Nausea _____

_____Other bodily pains _____

_____Paralysis _____

_____Phobias _____

_____Ringing in ears _____

_____Sexual indifference _____

_____Shaking or tremor _____

_____Spasms _____

_____Sudden weight fluctuation _____

_____Tics-verbal or motor _____

_____Trouble doing anything because felt bad _____

_____Unconsciousness _____

_____Urinary retention _____

_____Visual blurring _____

_____Vomiting _____

_____Vomiting all nine months of pregnancy _____

_____Weakness _____

_____Weight loss _____

Other Medical Problems:

_____Alcoholism _____

_____Chronic illness _____

_____Diagnosed illness _____

_____Diagnosed mental disorder _____

_____Drug addiction _____

_____Emotional abuse _____

_____Physical abuse _____

_____Sexual abuse _____

NEW MIND NEUROFEEDBACK CENTER
TRAINING SESSION REPORT

Client _____   Date _____

Clinician _____   Time _____ A.M. ___ P.M. ___

                                            Inter-protocol # _____

Presenting problem status   ### Status Notes   Total sessions # _____

Sleep   Headaches _____

Awareness of dreams   Focus _____

Nightmares   Concentration _____

Boundary clarification   Attention _____

Reduced emotional reactivity   Memory _____

Enhanced calmness   Moodiness _____

Energy level   Irritability _____

(Protocol) Screen Name _____

Baseline 1   ### Baseline 2

Site _____ Notes_____   Site _____ Notes_____

(Freq)	EO	EC		(Freq)	EO	EC
_____	F1 ____	F1 ____		_____	F1 ____	F1 ____
_____	F2 ____	F2 ____		_____	F2 ____	F2 ____
_____	F3 ____	F3 ____		_____	F3 ____	F3 ____
_____	F4 ____	F4 ____		_____	F4 ____	F4 ____

Trial 1   ### Trial 2   ### Trial 3   ### Trial 4

Notes _____   Notes _____   Notes _____   Notes _____

Protocol _____   Protocol _____   Protocol _____   Protocol _____

Site _____   Site _____   Site _____   Site _____

Time _____   Time _____   Time _____   Time _____

EO EC   EO EC   EO EC   EO EC

VE: L ____ R ____   VE: L ____ R ____   VE: L ____ R ____   VE: L ____ R ____

Goals   ### Goals   ### Goals   ### Goals

F1 F2 F3 F4   F1 F2 F3 F4   F1 F2 F3 F4   F1 F2 F3 F4

μV __ __ __ __ μV __ __ __ __ μV __ __ __ __ μV __ __ __ __

% __ __ __ __   % __ __ __ __   % __ __ __ __   % __ __ __ __

L   R   L   R   L   R   L   R

(Freq) Trial 1 Results   (Freq) Trial 2 Results   (Freq) Trial 3 Results   (Freq) Trial 4 Results

____ F1 ___ ___   ____ F1 ___ ___   ____ F1 ___ ___   ____ F1 ___ ___

____ F2 ___ ___   ____ F2 ___ ___ .   ____ F2 ___ ___   ____ F2 ___ ___

____ F3 ___ ___   ____ F3 ___ ___   ____ F3 ___ ___   ____ F3 ___ ___

____ F4 ___ ___   ____ F4 ___ ___   ____ F4 ___ ___   ____ F4 ___ ___

Session Notes:

NEW MIND NEUROFEEDBACK CENTER
SYMPTOM CHECKLIST

At the beginning of each session, use this checklist to help evaluate and track your progress. Rate yourself. On a scale of 1 to 10 regarding each of the items below, use 1 as low, little, or poor, and use 10 as high, a lot, or excellent. Use a marker to trace over each dotted line to create a bar graph.

	1 Lo	5 Average	10 Hi
Concentration			
Short-term Memory			
Quality of Sleep			
Appetite			
Motivation/Energy			
Positive Moods			
Patience			
Asserteness			
Restlessness			
Worry/Negative Thinking			
Negative Mood*			
Negative Emotions			
Pain/Physical Discomfort			
Fatigue			
Irritability			
Impulsivity**			

*An emotion lasts 20 minutes to an hour, a mood lasts several hours, days, or weeks.

**Impulsivity includes disorganization, foot in mouth, impulse buying, blowing up at people, and so forth.

This test is also available on our website and clients can fill it out from home: https://newmindmaps.com/

NEW MIND Neurofeedback Center
SAMPLE PROTOCOL WORKSHEET

Date _____ Patient verbalizes awareness of protocol change _____ _____

Clinician's initials   *Patient initials*

Client _____

Protocol _____
EO   EC
Rational _____

Sx changes_____
Client-specific indicators

_____   _____

_____   _____

_____   _____

Date _____ Patient verbalizes awareness of protocol change _____ _____

Clinician's initials   *Patient initials*

Client _____

Protocol _____
EO   EC
Rational _____

Sx changes_____
Client-specific indicators

_____   _____

_____   _____

_____   _____

Alpha-theta training involves placing you (the client) in a twilight state between waking and consciousness. In this state, you may recover lost memories and feelings associated with traumatic events or key points in your life. At New Mind Neurofeedback Center (NMNC), we deal immediately with these issues through EMDR to reduce emotional turmoil and discomfort associated with such phenomena. However, mild irritability and anxiety can often continue for several days. If you have serious traumas, you may experience discomfort for several weeks.

Be sure to keep your therapist abreast of feelings associated with your training and alert your therapist to any problems you are having. It is not advisable to stop treatment due to such discomfort; however, if you decide to discontinue treatment, NMNC will not be held liable for the consequences. Be prepared to take days off from work if necessary. If you have an issue with alcohol, you should be aware that drinking during training may affect you in unusual ways and any contact with alcohol could result in rashes and/or flu-like symptoms.

Physiological changes can also alter your sensitivity to various foods. It is possible that you will experience changes in your personality as well, which can affect your personal relationships and occupation. Furthermore, you are advised that failure to follow recommendations or to show up for regular training sessions may result in reduced effectiveness of training.

I have read and understand the above and freely consent to participate in the training sessions in full understanding of the ramifications and consequences. I, further, understand that NMNC cannot be held liable for the above negative consequences should I fail to follow their recommendations during the training period.

Signed: _____ Date: _____

Name: _____
     (First)   (Middle In.)   (Last)

Appendix E: Suggested Reading List

NEUROFEEDBACK

History and Technique

Cade, Maxwell C., & Coxhead, Nona. (1989). *The Awakened Mind: Biofeedback and the Development of Higher States of Awareness*. Dorset, England: Element Books.

> Cade was one the first to use EEG to guide changes in behavior and consciousness. He was among the first to identify key features of the EEG relating to meditative states. A classic in the field.

Femi, Les, & Robbins, Jim. (2008). *The Open-Focus Brain: Harnessing the Power of Attention to Heal Mind and Body*. Boston, MA: Shambhalla/Trumpeter.

> Les Femi understands attention and how it relates to consciousness better than almost anyone out there. His workshops on open focus attention are a revelation about how we use attention without knowing it. His specialty area is 4-channel coherence training, and he has been doing it for decades. Jim Robbins, a science writer for the *New York Times* who personally explored many of the paradigms of neurofeedback, was especially attracted to this approach.

Green, E. E., & Green, A. M. (1977). *Beyond Biofeedback*. San Francisco: Delacorte.

> Elmer pioneered this whole field and created his own equipment and methods. We still have not followed through in replicating the research and equipment he devised decades ago. This book is a fascinating story of his journey and a must-read for anyone in the field.

Robbins, Jim. (2000). *A Symphony in the Brain*. New York: Grove Hills.

> This is the book you give to all your clients who want to know more about neurofeedback.

Soutar, R. & Crane, A. (2000). *Mindfitness Training: Neurofeedback and the Process*. New York: iUniverse.

> Discusses a lot of the theoretical underpinnings of peak performance training — not a how-to manual.

Soutar, R. (2006). *The Automatic Self: Transformation & Transcendence through Brainwave Training.* New York: I Universe.

> Written for the general public, this book explicates its theme on many levels and is a favorite of clinicians while at the same time a mysterious waste of time to the technical people in the field. It reviews the profound implications of the manner in which the nervous system manages information and behavior. It then discusses how neurofeedback can fundamentally alter the consequences of this human dilemma. Although the premise is not new and may seem simple and obvious, clearly most people have not understood it well or the world would be a different place.

Wise, Anna. (1997). *The High Performance Mind.* New York: G.P. Putnam's Sons.

> Anna's work has been a great unacknowledged contribution to the field and is essential for anyone planning to do deep states training with neurofeedback.

Applications

Budzynski, T. H., Budzynski, H. K., Evans, J. R., & Abarbanel, A. (Eds.). (2009). *Introduction to Quantitative EEG and Neurofeedback, Second Edition: Advanced Theory and Applications.* Burlington, MA: Elsevier Publications.

Evans, J. R. (Ed.). (2007). *Handbook of Neurofeedback: Dynamics and Clinical Applications.* New York: The Hawthorne Medical Press.

Hill, R. W., & Castro, E. (2002). *Getting Rid of Ritalin: How Neurofeedback Can Successfully Treat Attention Deficit Disorder Without Drugs.* Charlottesville, VA: Hampton Roads Publishing Co., Inc.

Larson, S. (2006). *The Healing Power of Neurofeedback: The Revolutionary LENS Technique for Restoring Optimal Brain Function.* Rochester, VT: Healing Arts Press.

Othmer, S. (2008). *Protocol Guide for Neurofeedback Clinicians.* Woodland Hills, CA: EEG Info.

Swingle, P. G. (2008). *Biofeedback for the Brain: How Neurotherapy Effectively Treats Depression, ADHD, Autism, and More.* NJ: Rutgers University Press.

Thompson, M., & Thompson, L. (2003). *The Neurofeedback Book: An Introduction to Basic Concepts in Applied Psychophysiology.* Wheat Ridge, CO: AAPB.

Heavier and More Clinically Oriented

Demos, John. (2005). *Getting Started With Neurofeedback.* New York: W.W. Norton & Company.

> When John called me up and said he was planning to write an easy-to-read introduction to neurofeedback for clinicians entering the field, I sent him *Doing*

Neurofeedback and pointed him in the direction of some good research. He went to scads of workshops by everyone in the field and took copious notes. The result is this highly proclaimed and excellent book that every practitioner should read before he or she lifts an electrode.

Neuroscience

Some good basic reading on neurocognitive science that applies to clinical neurofeedback.

Cozolino, Louis (2002). *The Neuroscience of Psychotherapy: Building and Rebuilding The Human Brain.* New York: Norton.

> One of the best books written on the relationship between talk therapy and resulting changes in neurophysiology.

Demasio, Antonio. (1994). *Descartes' Error: Emotion, Reason, and the Human Brain.* New York: Avon Books.

> Demasio was among the first to define how the emotional brain impacts the frontal lobes in terms of executive function and social behavior. A very readable text.

Demasio, Antonio. (1999). *The Feeling of What Happens.* New York: Harcourt Brace.

> A very good sequel to *Descartes' Error* on consciousness and self-construction.

Goleman, D. (1995). *Emotional Intelligence.* New York: Bantam Books.

> This book was the first definitive book explaining the important role of emotion and limbic structures in social behavior. This is a must-read for all neurotherapy clinicians.

Le Doux, Joseph. (1996). *The Emotional Brain: The Mysterious Underpinnings of Emotional Life.* New York: Simon & Schuster.

> Le Doux is an excellent writer and able to make complex topics simple to understand. He is a leading researcher in fear conditioning and how it relates to anxiety and PTSD. The material here will provide you with an excellent basis for better understanding the anatomy and physiology of anxiety.

Le Doux, Joseph. (2002). *The Synaptic Self: How Our Brains Became Who We Are.* New York: Viking.

A good sequel to *The Emotional Brain.*

Posner, Michael I., & Raichle, Marcus E. (1997) *Images of Mind.* New York: Scientific American Library.

This was very popular reading at ISNR years ago and still stands up well today. It provides excellent pictures and diagrams and covers the topic of attention in a detailed and informative manner that is very useful to neurofeedback clinicians and individuals involved in QEEG and MiniQ.

Schore, A. N. (1994). *Affect Regulation and the Origin of the Self: The Neurobiology of Emotional Development.* Hillsdale, NJ: Lawrence Erlbaum Associates.

Schores's book is acknowledged universally as the definitive treatise on the topic of trauma and how it impacts development, socialization, and emotional functioning.

Schwartz, Jeffrey M., & Begley, Sharon. (2002). *The Mind and The Brain.* New York: Harper Collins.

This is one of the best books on OCD we have read. It explains the disorder right down to the "worry circuit" the authors have identified as the source of obsessive thinking. It is also an excellent book on the brain in general as well as providing interesting theoretical ideas toward resolving the mind-brain problem.

Brain Functions (Heavy Reading)

Crosson, Bruce. (1992). *Subcortical Functions in Language and Memory.* New York: The Guilford Press.

Those interested in memory and language function will find all the details regarding structures and networks that are associated. Be prepared for a complex and dry rendition that raises more questions than it answers.

Chow, T. W., & Cummings, J. L. (1998). Frontal-Subcortical Circuits. In Bruce L. Miller & Jeffrey L. Cummings (Eds.), *The Human Frontal Lobes* (pp. 3-44). New York: The Guilford Press.

For those interested in finding out every little detail about how executive function operates and drive the rest of the brain, this is the book. This text reviews all of the structures and networks as well as most of the MRI research regarding brain function.

Kaplan, G. B., & Hammer, R. P. (2002). *Brain Circuitry and Signaling in Psychiatry: Basic Science and Implications*. Washington, DC: American Psychiatric Publishing.

> You definitely want this one for your bookshelf. It covers many of the major disorders and the networks identified as being involved as well as a good review of the research regarding the impact of drugs on these disorders. Well written and easy to understand with lots of diagrams and pictures to help.

Electrophysiology (Heavy Reading)

Books that are pertinent to QEEG and fairly heavy reading - 'nuff said.

Nunez, Paul L. (Ed.). (1995). *Neocortical Dynamics and Human EEG Rhythms*. New York: Oxford University Press.

Lubar, J. (2004). *Quantitative Electroencephalographic Analysis (QEEG) Databases for Neurotherapy: Description, Validation, and Application*. Binghamton, NY: The Haworth Medical Press.

Entrainment

Siever, Dave. (1999). *The Rediscovery of Audio-Visual Entrainment Technology*. Edmonton, Alberta, Canada: Comptronic Devices Limited.

> If you are interested in entrainment, this is the book to get. Period.

General

Amen, D. G. (2001). *Healing ADD: The Breakthrough Program that Allows You to See and Heal the 6 Types Of ADD*. New York: Berkley Books.

Arntz, W., Chasse, B., & Vicente, M. (2005). *What the Bleep Do We Know: Discovering the Endless Possibilities for Altering Your Everyday Reality*. Deerfield Beach, FL: Health Communications, Inc.

Begley, S. (2007). *Train Your Mind, Change Your Brain: How a New Science Reveals Our Extraordinary Potential to Transform Ourselves*. New York: Ballentine Books.

Campbell, D. (1997). *The Mozart Effect: Tapping the Power of Music to Heal the Body, Strengthen the Mind, and Unlock the Creative Spirit*. New York: Avon Books.

Gladwell, M. (2005). *Blink: The Power of Thinking Without Thinking*. New York: Little, Brown and Co.

Lipton, B. (2005). *The Biology of Belief: Unleashing the Power of Consciousness, Matter, and Miracles*. Santa Rosa, CA: Mountain of Love/Elite Books.

Moyers, B. (1993). *Healing and the Mind*. New York: Doubleday.

Promislow, S. (2005). *Making the Brain Body Connection: A Playful Guide to Releasing Mental, Physical, & Emotional Blocks to Success*. Vancouver, BC, Canada: Enhanced Learning & Integration, Inc.

Stein, P., & Kendall, J. (2004). *Psychological Trauma and the Developing Brain: Neurologically Based Interventions for Troubled Children*. New York: The Hawthorne Maltreatment and Trauma Press.

Steinberg, M. S., & Othmer, S. (2004). *ADD - The 20-Hour Solution: Training Minds to Concentrate and Self-Regulate Naturally without Medication*. Bandon, OR: Robert D. Reed Publishers.

Ziegler, D. (2002). *Traumatic Experience and the Brain: A Handbook for Understanding and Treating Those Traumatized as Children*. Phoenix, AZ: Acacia Publishing.

Neuroscience & the Brain

Amen, D. G. (2005). *Making a Good Brain Great*. New York: Three Rivers Press.

Amen, D. G. (1998). *Change Your Brain, Change Your Life: The Breakthrough Program for Conquering Anxiety, Depression, Obsessiveness, Anger and Impulsiveness*. New York: Three Rivers Press.

Braverman, E. R. (2004). *The Edge Effect: Achieve Total Health and Longevity with the Balanced Brain Advantage.* New York: Sterling Publishing Co.

De Haan, M., & Gunnar, M. R. (2009). *Handbook of Developmental Social Neuroscience*. New York: Guilford Press.

Dispenza, J. (2007). *Evolve Your Brain: The Science of Changing Your Mind*. Deerfield Beach, FL: Health Communications, Inc.

Katz, L. C., & Rubin, M. (1999). *Keep Your Brain Alive*. New York: Workman Publishing Co.

Kotulak, R. (1996). *Inside the Brain: Revolutionary Discoveries of How the Mind Works*. Kansas City, MO: Andrews McMeel Publishing.

Schiffer, F. (1998). *Of Two Minds: The Revolutionary Science of Dual Brain Psychology*. New York: Free Press.

Schore, A. N. (1994) *Affect Regulation and the Origin of the Self: The Neurobiology of Emotional Development*. Hillsdale, NJ: Erlbaum.

Siegel, D. J. (1999). *The Developing Mind: Toward a Neurobiology of Interpersonal Experience*. New York: Guilford Press.

Siegel, D. J. (2007). *The Mindful Brain: Reflection and Attunement in the Cultivation of Well-Being*. New York: W. W. Norton & Company.

Teicher, M. H. (2002). Scars that Won't Heal: The Neurobiology of Child Abuse. *Scientific American, 286*(3), 68-75.

APPENDIX F: REFERENCES

There is a great deal more research available, and we recommend reading every issue of the *Journal of Neurotherapy* going back to issue one. Corey Hammond has a wonderful listing of research on each disorder published in the *Journal of Neurotherapy,* 2001, Volume 5, Numbers 1/2.

A great deal of this book's lead author's information also comes from informal conversations at conferences, workshops, and meetings with the individuals cited. These references are cited as "personal communication" and are too numerous to identify individually by date.

Alper, K. R., Prichep, L. S., Kowalik, S., Rosenthal, M. S., & John, E. R. (1998). Persistent QEEG abnormality in crack cocaine users at 6 months of drug abstinence. *Neuropsychopharmacology, 19,* 1-9.

Alstott, J., Breakspear, M., Hagmann, P., Cammoun, L., & Sporns, O. (2009, June 12). Modeling the impact of lesions in the human brain. *PLoS Computational Biology, 5*(6), e1000408.

American Academy of Experts in Taumatic Stress, Inc. (1998). *The American Academy of Experts in Traumatic Stress.* Retrieved May 1, 2010, from the Peniston-Kulkosky Brainwave Neurofeedback Therapeutic Protocol: The Future Psychotherapy for Alcoholism/PTSD/Behavioral Medicine: http://www.aaets.org/arts/art47.htm

Anderson, P., & Anderson, S. A. (1968). *Physiological aasis of the alpha rhythm.* New York, NY: Appleton Century Crofts.

Amen, D. G. (1998). *Change your brain, change your life.* New York, NY: Random House.

Association for Applied Psychophysiology and Biofeedback, Inc. (2008). Retrieved May 1, 2010, from News & Media Coverage: http://www.aapb.org/news.html

Baehr, E., Rosenfeld, J. P., & Baehr, R. (1997). The clinical use of an alpha asymmetry protocol in the neurofeedback treatment of depression: Two case studies. *Journal of Neurotherapy, 3,* 12-23.

Bassett, D. S., Meyer-Lindenberg, A., Achard, S., Duke, T., & Bullmore, E. (2006). Adaptive reconfiguration of fractal small-world human brain functional networks. *Proceedings of the National Academy of Sciences, 103*(51), 19518-19523.

Beck, A. T. (1979). *Cognitive therapy and the emotional disorders.* Cleveland, OH: Meridian.

Begley, S. (2007). *Train your mind, change your brain: How a new science reveals our extraordinary potential to transform ourselves.* New York, NY: Ballentine Books.

Brain Paint. (2007). *Bill Scott's biography sketch.* Retrieved May 1, 2010, from Brain Paint: http://www.brainpaint.com/index_files/aboutbillscott.htm

Brown, V. W. (1995). Neurofeedback and Lyme's disease: A clinical application of the five-phase model of CNS functional transformation and integration. *Journal of Neurotherapy, 1*(2), 60-73.

Brown, V. (2010). *Author page.* Retrieved May 1, 2010, from Future Health: http://www.futurehealth.org/populum/authors_productpage.php?sid=418

Buckner, R. L., Andrews-Hanna, J. R., & Schacter, D. L. (2008). The brain's default network: Anatomy, function, and relevance to disease. *Annals of the New York Academy of Sciences, 11*(24), 1-38.

Buzsaki, G. (2006). *Rhythms of the brain.* New York, NY: Oxford University Press.

Chabot, R. J., Prichep, L., & Flavia, M. D. (2005). The role of quantitative electroencephalography in child and adolescent psychiatric disorders. *Child and Adolescent Psychiatric Clinics of North America, 14,* 21-53.

Chabot, R. (1998). Quantitative EEG profiles and LORETA imaging of children with attention deficit and learning disorders. Presentation at 1998 SNR Conference.

Changeux, J. P. (1985). *Neuronal man: The biology of mind.* Princeton, NJ: Princeton University Press.

Chow, T. W., & Cummings, J. L. (1998). Frontal-subcortical circuits. In B. L. Miller & J. L. Cummings (Eds.), *The human frontal lobes: Functions and disorders* (pp. 3-26). New York, NY: The Guilford Press.

Cohen, G., Johnston, R. A., & Plunkett, K. (2000). *Exploring cognition: damaged brains and neural networks: Readings in cognitive neuropsychology and connectionist modeling.* East Sussex, UK: Psychology Press.

Crane, A., & Soutar, R. (2000). *Mindfitness training: Neurofeedback and the process.* Lincoln, NE: Writer's Club Press.

Criswell, E. (1995). *Biofeedback & somatics: Toward personal evolution.* Novato, CA: Freeperson Press.

Crossen, B. (1992). *Subcortical functions in language and memory.* New York, NY: The Guilford Press.

Evans, J. R. (1999). *Handbook of neurofeedback: Dynamics and clinical applications.* New York, NY: The Hawthorne Medical Press.

Evans, J. R., & Abarbanel, A. (1999). *Introduction to quantitative EEG and neurofeedback.* San Diego, CA: Academic Press.

Duffy, F. H., Iyer, V. G., & Surwillo, W. W. (1989). *Clinical electroencephalography and topographic brain mapping: Technology and practice.* New York, NY: Springer-Vrlag.

Dyro, F. M. (1989). *The EEG handbook.* Boston, MA: Little Brown Company.

Davidson, R. J. (1995). Cerebral asymmetry, emotion, and affective style. In R. Davidson, & K. Hugdahl, *Brain asymmetry* (pp. 361-387). Cambridge, MA: MIT Press.

Davidson, R. J., Jackson, D. C., & Kalin, N. H. (2000). Emotion, plasticity, context, and regulation: Perspectives from affective neuroscience. *Psychological Bulletin, 126*(6), 890-909.

DeBeus, R., Ball, J. D., DeBeus, M. E., & Herrington, R. (2003). *Attention training with ADHD children: Preliminary findings in a double blind placebo controlled study.* Presented at the International Society for Neuronal Regulation Annual Conference, Houston, Texas.

Demasio, A. (1994). *Descartes' error: Emotion, reason, and the human brain.* New York, NY: Avon Books.

Demasio, A. (1999). *The feeling of what happens.* New York, NY: Harcourt Brace.

Demos, J. M. (2005). *Getting started with neurofeedback.* New York, NY: W. W. Norton & Company.

Diamond, M. C., Scheibel, A. B., & Lawrence, M. (1985). *The human brain coloring book.* New York, NY: Harper Collins.

Drevets, W. C., Price, J. L., & Jr., J. R. (1997). Subgenual prefrontal cortex abnormalities in mood disorders. *Nature, 386,* 824-827.

Femi, L. G. (1978). EEG biofeedback, multichannel synchrony training, and attention. In A. Sugarman, *Expanding dimensions of consciousness.* New York, NY: Springer Verlag. pp 152-182

Fitzgerald, M. J., & Folan-Curran, J. (2002). *Clinical neuroanatomy and related neuroscience.* New York, NY: W. B. Saunders.

Freeman, W. J., Ahlfors, S. P., & Menon, V. (2009). Combining fMRI with EEG and MEG in order to relate patterns of brain activity to cognition. *International Journal of Psychophysiology, 73*(1), 43-52.

Friedemann, P., Eulitz, C., Pantev, C., Lutzenberger, W., Elbert, T., Preissl, H., et al. (1994). Brain rhythms, cell assemblies and cognition: Evidence from the processing of words and pseudowords. *Psycoloquy, 5,* 48.

Gunkelman, J. (1998). Drug exposure and EEG/QEEG findings. *Future Health Presentation Handout.* Future Health. Palm Springs, California. Available through the authors

Gunkleman, J. (1999). QEEG patterns, sources and NF interventions. *SNR Workshop.* Myrtle Beach, Florida

Gläscher, J., Tranel, D., Paul, L. K., Rudrauf, D., Rorden, C., Hornaday, A., et al. (2009). *Lesion mapping of cognitive abilities linked to intelligence.* Retrieved May 2, 2010, from Science Direct: http://www.sciencedirect.com/science/article/pii/S1053811909706858

Green, E. (1992). Alpha-theta brainwave training: Instrumental vipassana? *Montreal Symposium.* Montreal, Canada.

Green, E. E., Green, A. M., & Walters, D. E. (1970). Voluntary control of internal states: Psychological and physiological. *Journal of Transpersonal Psychology, 2*(1), 1-26.

Green, E., & Green, A. M. (1977). *Beyond biofeedback.* San Francisco, CA: Delacorte.

Hughes, J. R., & John, E. R. (1999). Conventional and quantitative electroencephalography in psychiatry. *Journal of Neuropsychiatry and Clinical Neuroscience, 11*(2), 190-208.

Hughes, S. W., & Cruneli, V. (2005). Thalamic mechanisms of EEG alpha rhythms and their pathological implications. *The Neuroscientist, 11*(4), 357-372.

Hagmann, P., Cammoun, L., Gigandet, X., Meuli, R., Honey, C. J., Wedeen, V. J., et al. (2008). Mapping the structural core of human cerebral cortex. *PLoS Biology, 6*(7), 1479-1493.

Hammond, C., & Kirk, L. (2008). First do no harm: Adverse effects and the need for practice standards in neurofeedback. *Journal of Neurotherapy, 12*(1), 79-88.

Hammond, D., Walker, J., Hoffman, D., Lubar, J., Trudeau, D., Gurnee, R., et al. (2004). Standards for the use of quantitative electroencephalography (qeeg) in neurofeedback: A position paper of the International Society for Neuronal Regulation. *Journal of Neurotherapy, 8*(1), 5-27.

Hartmann, T. (1993). *Attention deficit disorder: A different perception.* Grass Valley, CA: Underwood Books.

Homan, R. W., Herman, J., & Purdy, P. (1987). Cerebral Location of International 10-20 System Electrode Placement. *Electroencephalography and Clinical Neurophysiology, 66*(4), 376-382.

John, E. R., Karmel, B., Corning, W., Easton, P., D., B., Ahn, H., et al. (1977). Neurometrics: Neurometrical taxonomy identifies different profiles of brain functions within groups of behaviorally similar people. *Science, 196,* 1393-1410.

John, E. R., Prichep, L. S., Fridman, J., & Easton, P. (1988). Neurometrics: Computer assisted differential diagnosis of brain dysfunctions. *Science, 293*, 162-169.

Johnstone, J. (2001). Effect of antidepressant medications on the EEG. *Journal of Neurotherapy, 5*(4), 93-97.

Kaplan, G. B., & Hammer, R. P. (2002). *Brain circuitry and signaling in psychiatry: Basic science and implications.* Washington, DC: American Psychiatric Publishing.

Kolb, B., & Whishaw, I. Q. (1996). *Fundamentals of human neuropsychology* (4th ed.). Alberta, Canada: University of Lethbridge/Worth Publishers.

Lubar, J. F. (1991). Discourse on the development of EEG diagnostics and biofeedback for attention-deficit hyperactivity disorders. *Biofeedback & Self-Regulation, 16*(3), 201-225.

Lubar, J. F. (1995). Neurofeedback for the management of attention deficit/hyperactivity disorders. In M. S. Schwartz, *Biofeedback: A practitioner's guide* (pp. 493-522). New York, NY: Guilford.

Lubar, J. F. (1997). Neocortical dynamics: implications for understanding the role of neurofeedback and related techniques for the enhancement of attention. *Applied Psychophysiology and Biofeedback, 22*, 11-126.

Lubar, J. F., & Lubar, J. (1999). Neurofeedback assessment and treatment for attention deficit/hyperactivity disorders. In J. R. Evans & A. Abarbanel (Eds.), *Introduction to quantitative EEG and neurofeedback* (pp. 243-310). New York, NY: Academic Press.

Larson, S. (2006). *The healing power of neurofeedback: The revoluntionary lens technique for restoring optimal brain function.* Rochester, NY: Healing Arts Press.

Le Doux, J. (1996). *The emotional brain: The mysterious underpinnings of emotional life.* New York, NY: Simon & Schuster.

McCormick, D. A. (1999). Are thalamocortical rhythms the Rosetta Stone of a subset of neurological disorders? *Mature Medicine, 5*(12), 1349-1351.

McEwen, B. (1987). Influence of hormones and neuroactive substances on immune function. In C. W. Cotman, *The neuro-immune-endocrine connection.* New York, NY: Raven Press. pp 33-47.

McIntosh, A. R., & Korostil, M. (2008). Interpretation of neuroimaging data based on network concepts. *Brain Imaging and Behavior*, 264-269.

Monstra, V. J., Lynn, S., Linden, M., Lubar, J. F., Gruzelier, J., & Vaque, T. J. (2005). Electroencephalographic biofeedback in the treatment of ADHD. *Applied Psychophysiology and Biofeedback, 30*(2), 95-114.

Montgomery, D. D., Robb, J., Dwyer, K. V., & Gontkovsky, S. T. (1998). Single channel QEEG amplitudes in a bright, normal young adult sample. *Journal of Neurotherapy*, 1-7.

Moss, D. (1998). *Humanistic and transpersonal psychology: A historical and biographical sourcebook.* Retrieved May 1, 2010, from Biofeedback, Mind-Body Medicine, and the Higher Limits of Human Nature: http://nealmiller.org/?p=94

Nunez, P. (1995). *Neocortical dynamics and human EEG rhythms.* New York, NY: Oxford Unversity Press.

Niedermeyer, E., & Silva, F. H. (1999). *Electroencephalography: Basic principles, clinical applications and related fields* (4th ed.). New York, NY: Lippincott Williams & Eilkins.

Ochs, L. (2010). *Author's page.* Retrieved May 1, 2010, from Future Health: http://www.futurehealth.org/populum/authors_productpage.php?sid=424

Othmer, S. (2008). *Protocol guide for neurofeedback clinicians.* Woodland Hills, CA: EEG Info.

Othmer, S. (1994). Training syllabus. *EEG Spectrum, 1.*

Othmer, S., Othmer, S. F., & Kaiser, D. A. (1999). EEG biofeedback: An emerging model for its global efficacy. In J. R. Evans, & A. Abarbanel, *Introduction to quantitative EEG and neurofeedback* (pp. 243-310). New York, NY: Academic Press.

Pascual-Marqui, R. D. (2007, November 9). *Instantaneous and lagged measurements of linear and nonlinear dependence between groups of multivariate time series: Frequency decomposition.* Retrieved August 16, 2010, from Arsiv.org: http://arsiv.org/abs/0711.1455

Patent Storm. (2010). *Electrode locator - US Patent 5518007 Description.* Retrieved May 1, 2010, from Patent Storm: http://www.patentstorm.us/patents/5518007/description.html

Peniston, B. G., & Kulkosky, P. J. (1989). Alpha-theta brainwave training and beta-endorphin levels in alcoholics. *Alcohol, 13,* 271-279.

Plutchik, R. (1980). *Emotion: A psychoevolutionary synthesis.* New York, NY: Harper Collins.

Posner, M. I., & Raichle, M. E. (1997). *Images of mind.* New York, NY: Scientific American Library.

Suffin, S. C., & Emory, W. H. (1995). Neurometric subgroups in attentional and affective disorders and their association with pharmacotherapeutic outcome. *Clinical Electroencephalography, 26,* 76-83.

Swingle, P. C. (2008). *Biofeedback for the brain: How neurotherapy effectively treats depression, ADHD, autism, and more.* New Jersey: Rutgers University Press.

Schwartz, J. M., & Begley, S. (2002). *The Mind & the brain: Neuroplasticity and the power of mental force.* New York, NY: Regan Books.

Schacter, S., & Singer, J. E. (1962). Cognitive, social, and physiological determinants of emotional state. *Psychological Review, 69*(5), 379-399.

Schiffer, F. (1998). *Of two minds: The revolutionary science of dual brain psychology.* New York, NY: Free Press.

Schmahmann, J. D., & Pandya, D. N. (2006). *Fiber pathways of the brain.* New York, NY: Oxford University Press.

Schore, A. N. (1994). *Affect regulation and the origin of the self: The neurobiology of emotional development.* Hillsdale, NJ: Lawrence Erlbaum Associates.

Scott, W. C., Brod, T. M., Siderhof, S., Kaiser, D., & Sagan, M. (2002). Type-specific EEG biofeedback improves residential substance abuse treatment. *American Psyciatric Association Conference.*

Scott, W., Kaiser, D., Othmer, S., & Sideroff, S. I. (2005). Effects of an EEG biofeedback protocol on a mixed substance abusing population. *American Journal of Drug and Alcohol Abuse, 31*(3), 455-469.

Siever, D. (1999). *The rediscovery of audio-visual entrainment technology.* Alberta, Canada: Comptronic Devices Limited. Edmonton, Alberta, Canada

Sheer, D. E. (1976). Focused arousal and 40 Hz EEG. In D. J. Bakker, & R. M. Knights, *The neurophysiology of learning disorders.* Baltimore, MD: University Park Press. pp 71-87

Sherlin, L., & Congedo, M. (2005). Obsessive compulsive disorder localized using low resolution electromagnetic brain tomography (LORETA). *Neuroscience Letters, 387*(2), 72-74.

Soutar, R. G. (2006). *The automatic self: Transformation and transcedence through brainwave training.* Lincoln, NE: iUniverse.

Soutar, R., & Crane, A. (2000). *Mindfitness training.* New York, NY: iUniverse.

Srinivasan, R., & Nunez, P. L. (2006). *Electric fields of the brain: The neurophysics of EEG.* New York, NY: Oxford University Press.

Sterman, M. B., & Bowersox, S. S. (1981). Sensorimotor electroencephalogram rhythmic activity: A functional gate mechanism. *Sleep, 4*(4), 408-422.

Sterman, M. B., & Mann, C. A. (1995). Concepts and applications of EEG analysis in aviation performance evaluation. *Biological Psychology, 40*, 115-130.

Sterman, M. B., Kaiser, D. A., & Veigel, B. (1966). Spectral analysis of event related EEG responses during short-term memory performance. *Brain Topography, 9*(1), 21-30.

Stien, P. T., & Kendall, J. (2004). *Psychological trauma and the developing brain: Neurologically based interventions for troubled children.* New York, NY: The Hawthorne Maltreatment and Trauma Press.

Streifel, S. (1995). Professional ethical behavior for providers of biofeedback. In M. S. Associates, *Biofeedback: A practitioner's guide* (pp. 685-705). New York, NY: The Guilford Press.

Striefel, S. (1989). A perspective on ethics. *Biofeedback, 17*(1), 21-22.

Ruden, R. A. (1997). *The craving brain: The biobalance approach to controlling addictions.* New York, NY: Harper Collins.

Ruden, R. R., & Byalick, M. (1997). *The craving brain: A bold new approach to breaking free from drug addiction, overeating, alcoholism, and gambling.* New York, NY: Harper Collins Books.

Robbins, J. (2000). *A symphony in the brain: The evolution of the new brain wave biofeedback.* New York, NY: Grove Press.

Rotter, J. R. (1990). Internal vs. external control of reinforcement. *American Psychologist*, 489-493.

Teicher, M. H. (2007). Childhood abuse, brain development and impulsivity. Keynote speech, Massachusetts Adolescent Sex Offender Coalition/Massachusetts Assocation for the Treatment of Sexual Abusers Joint Conference, April 7, Marlboro, MA.

Thatcher, R. W. (1998). Normative EEG databases and EEG biofeedback. *Journal of Neurotherapy, 2*(4), 8-39.

Thatcher, R. W., Walker, R. A., Biver, C. J., North, D. N., & Curtin, R. (2003). Quantitative EEG normative databases: Validation and clinical correlation. *Journal of Neurotherapy, 7*(3/4), 87-121.

Thatcher, R. W., Camacho, M., Salazar, A., Linden, C., Biver, C., & Clark, L. (1997). Quantitative MRI of the gray-white matter distribution in traumatic brain injury. *Journal of Neurotrauma, 14*, 1-14.

The Menninger Clinc. (2010). *History.* Retrieved May 1, 2010, from The Menninger Clinic: http://www.menningerclinic.com/about/Menninger-history.htm

Thompson, M., & Thompson, L. (2003). *The neurofeedback book: An introduction to basic concepts in applied psychophysiology.* Wheat Ridge, CO: AAPB.

Thornton, K. (2000). Rehabilitation of memory functioning in brain injured subject with EEG biofeedback. *Journal of Head Trauma Rehabilitation, 15*(6), 1285-1296.

Thorton, K., & Carmody, D. (2008). Efficacy of traumatic brain injury rehabilitation: Interventions of QEEG-guided biofeedback, computers, strategies, and medications. *Applied Psychophysiology and Biofeedback, 33*, 101-124.

Travis, T. A., Kondo, C. Y., & Knott, J. R. (1974). Parameters of eyes closed alpha enhancement. *Psychophysiology, 11*(6), 674-681.

Training & Research Institute, Inc. (2004). *The neurobiology of child abuse* [Poster]. Albuquerque, NM: Author. Retrieved from: http://trainingandresearch.com/58275.html

Walker, J. E., Charles, A., & Weber, R. K. (2002). Impact of QEEG-guided coherence training for patients with a mild closed head injury. *Journal of Neurotherapy, 6*(2), 31-43.

Watts, D. J. (2004). *Small worlds.* Princeton, NJ: Princeton University Press.

Wise, A. (1997). *The high performance mind.* New York, NY: G. P. Putham's Sons.

Ziegler, D. (2002). *Traumatic experience and the brain: A handbook for understanding and treating those traumatized as children.* Phoenix, AZ: Acacia Publishing.